LECTURE NOTES ON
GERIATRICS

DEDICATION

All hospital secretaries are wonderful;
but none nearly so wonderful as Pam
who runs the department so smoothly.
All wives are marvellous;
but Sally, Lilas and Sue
are especially so,
and we dedicate this edition
to these four people
who have helped us so enormously

LECTURE NOTES ON
GERIATRICS

NICHOLAS CONI
MA, FRCP

WILLIAM DAVISON
TD, OStJ, MA, FRCP(E)

STEPHEN WEBSTER
MD, MRCP

Consultant Physicians
in Geriatric Medicine
Addenbrooke's Hospital
and Associate Lecturers in the
Faculty of Clinical Medicine
University of Cambridge

FOREWORD BY

SIR JOHN BUTTERFIELD
OBE, MD, DM, FRCP
Regius Professor of Physic
University of Cambridge
Master of Downing College, Cambridge

THIRD EDITION

BLACKWELL SCIENTIFIC PUBLICATIONS

OXFORD LONDON EDINBURGH

BOSTON PALO ALTO MELBOURNE

©1977, 1980, 1988 by
Blackwell Scientific Publications
Editorial offices:
Osney Mead, Oxford OX2 0EL
(Orders: Tel. 0865-240201)
8 John Street, London WC1N 2ES
23 Ainslie Place, Edinburgh EH3 6AJ
Three Cambridge Center, Suite 208
    Cambridge, MA 02142, USA
667 Lytton Avenue, Palo Alto
    California 94301, USA
107 Barry Street, Carlton
    Victoria 3053, Australia

First published 1977
Second edition 1980
Reprinted 1984, 1986
Third edition 1988

Photoset by Enset (Photosetting),
Midsomer Norton, Bath, Avon
Printed in Great Britain at
Billing and Sons Limited,
Worcester

DISTRIBUTORS

USA
    Year Book Medical Publishers
    35 East Wacker Drive
    Chicago, Illinois 60601
    (Orders: Tel. 312-726-9733)

Canada
    The C.V. Mosby Company
    5240 Finch Avenue East
    Scarborough, Ontario
    (Orders: Tel. 416-298-1588)

Australia
    Blackwell Scientific Publications
    (Australia) Pty Ltd
    107 Barry Street
    Carlton, Victoria 3053
    (Orders: Tel. 03-347-0300)

British Library
Cataloguing in Publication Data

Coni, Nicholas
    Lecture notes on geriatrics.—3rd ed.
    1. Geriatrics
    I. Title II. Davison, William, 1925–
    III. Webster, Stephen
    618.97   RC952

ISBN 0-632-02067-9

Contents

Contents

Foreword to the First Edition

I am very pleased to commend to students of British Medicine, of all ages, these 'Lecture Notes on Geriatrics'.

The authors are a close-knit team providing the regular geriatric services to the elderly in and around Cambridge and, this being the inaugural year of the Clinical School, Coni, Davison and Webster are also accepting day-to-day responsibility for teaching their subject. Their book is being published soon after a Secretary of State for Health and Social Security has reported that over half the patients in acute hospital beds in England are over 65 years of age. So this crisp and compact manual is timely, and in my view timely for several other good reasons.

Good medical care and teamwork

First, the authors remind us that we should consider the whole patient and indicate why this is particularly important in geriatric cases. This assertion is not intended to imply that doctors and specialists in other fields are guilty of shortcoming in this fundamental aspect of good medical care. But it is a reminder to us all of an ideal to which we should re-dedicate ourselves with each new patient for whom we accept responsibility. Furthermore, valuable resources may be wasted if we do not adopt this holistic approach.

Second, the authors stress not only the resulting interdisciplinary nature of good care for so many medical cases, they also emphasize the role and responsibilities the medical profession must accept, integrating the various elements available. This integrative theme is particularly germane in the present climate following the recent reorganization of the National Health Service and points the way out of most of the organizational dilemmas which appear to beset us so much, so soon after that major upheaval.

Thirdly, and this it seems to me follows directly, current medical teamwork will rarely, perhaps never, be without social and personal health education components. In such circumstances geriatricians and general physicians must have much more contact than they did with those who work outside the hospital and clinic. Geriatricians have wider contacts and more experience in these matters than most of us and can help and guide us.

Regarding health education, I admit that there may be little health educational content for the elderly patient apart from teaching a general understanding of the use of any drugs prescribed—it is usually too late for much prevention—but there are often important health educational points for the family. Is this the kind of old age they want for themselves? Are they taking any steps now to secure a better, healthier old age than this elderly, ailing relative?

The clinical challenge of geriatrics

Until recently, the geriatric wards were regarded as burdensome, unrewarding and full of insoluble or unworthy clinical problems. The authors of this present book have brushed aside that image and presented the clinical picture of modern geriatric practice clearly and precisely. The chapters on diseases in the various body systems are excellent statements of today's realities with which medical students will be grappling from the moment they become pre-registration house officers. The coincidence of several disease processes in old age makes treatment more complex. This is a challenge to the doctor intent on good medical care for his elderly patients using the extensive therapeutic armoury of drugs.

The research and recruitment challenge of geriatrics

Undeniably, Medicine has its fashions. In the thirty years since I qualified there have been three waves of intellectual activity in clinical medicine which have attracted many, if not most, of the ablest minds, and three of which have had periods of much less appeal. There are no prizes for sorting the following alphabetical list into the appropriate groups: cardiology, general practice, geriatrics, immunology, psychiatry and renal medicine. There can be no doubt the intense interest in cardiology, renal medicine and immunology can be traced to research developments—Cournand's cardiac catheter, Richard's micropuncture of the renal glomerulus, McFarlane Burnet's immunological hypotheses.

It is my view that this present publication may excite students' interest and thus prepare the ground for the recruitment of able young investigators into the field of gerontology—a Cinderella subject at the moment, awaiting patiently the appearance of those research developments—which will be the vehicle for countless projects, Ph.D.'s and M.D. theses in the field and carry innumerable young people off to the glittering ball of professional success (and one not ending at midnight either).

Conclusions

To the intending readers of this book, I can give the following assurances. It gives an excellent and broad overview of the subject of geriatrics. It forms a well-balanced and useful basis for revision for students approaching their Finals, a revision which, through its multiple authorship, will almost certainly be rewarding for most practitioners and, I believe, many specialists. The style is lucid, the reading is easy and the subject matter practical: in how many other books does one find lecture notes for the general practitioner's own lecture to lay groups in the very first chapter?

But, most of all, I believe and hope this book may encourage more interest and recruitment into the field we must all practise now, and where, therefore, we must of necessity follow the masters, especially experienced and enthusiastic ones like Coni and his colleagues, Davison and Webster.

Cambridge, 1976   W. J. H. BUTTERFIELD

Preface to the
Third Edition

Geriatrics has come of age. The basic principles of geriatric medicine have become so widely appreciated and the frontiers of the subject so significantly advanced during the present decade that we have been gratified to find that a completely rewritten text is required. In order to avoid the temptation to expand we have deliberately pruned out virtually everything of a philosophical nature, and as much as possible of general medicine. The result is a much terser style with a greater reliance on tables and, we feel, a volume much more true to the aims and title of the 'Lecture Notes' series. We have also largely omitted drug doses and adverse effects—these can be looked up in the *British National Formulary* or *The Geriatric Prescriber**. It is our hope that this book will contain more information than the student needs for his finals and almost as much as the candidate requires for Membership or Diploma in Geriatric Medicine of the Royal College of Physicians of London.

The third edition is certainly far more comprehensive than its predecessors and we will be well rewarded if it wins as many friends throughout the world.

---

*Coni N.K., Davison W. & Reiss B. (1987) *The Geriatric Prescriber*. Blackwell Scientific Publications, Oxford.

Preface to the
First Edition

There is a danger that the current economic and political difficulties which beset the health and social services may blind us to the far greater crisis which is imminent. It is the vast and still growing burden of disease and disability in our increasing population of elderly people which threatens to overwhelm these services in the closing quarter of the century. The doctors and nurses of the future must be prepared both emotionally and intellectually to meet this challenge, whatever field of practice they subsequently enter. 'We are all geriatricians now' is a frequent claim, and indeed it is true that except for those specializing in paediatrics and obstetrics, all the professionals working in our health service will find they will spend the major part of their working lives looking after elderly patients. It is important therefore that they should have been taught to do it properly. General practice, general medicine and surgery, gynaecology, orthopaedics, urology, psychiatry and ophthalmology are all increasingly concerned with the diseases of old age. Fortunately, examiners for qualifying and higher examinations are beginning to realize this. Yet, there is still a comparative dearth of books on geriatric medicine aimed primarily at the undergraduate medical student.

It is intended that this book will help to fill the gap. In addition, it is hoped that it will be of value to general practitioners and general physicians who are being called upon more and more to provide a comprehensive geriatric service. Those chapters which are concerned with the organizational aspects of geriatric care are necessarily somewhat parochial in outlook. Nevertheless they may enable planners and medical administrators overseas to adopt what is best in the British system, and to avoid some of the pitfalls which have emerged. The clinical sections are also intended to help those studying for the membership examination, and the text has been designed to provide a source of information for nurses, health visitors and other professionals concerned with the care of the elderly. We also offer it as a practical guide to house physicians and registrars on joining the geriatric department. This book is in no sense a textbook of medicine, but is complementary to the many excellent ones available. In general, only those diseases showing a predilection for old age, or presenting special features in old age, are considered in any detail. Many other conditions which affect old and young alike are therefore only mentioned cursorily or are omitted altogether. To facilitate revision each chapter is intended to be reasonably complete. This inevitably leads to a certain amount of repetition, but repetition is an essential part of the learning process.

Furthermore, many of the ethical and logistic problems which beset us are left unanswered because they are at present unanswerable. We very much hope that our readers will be stimulated into thinking for themselves about the difficult questions raised by the demography of ageing and into providing some of the solutions.

Finally, geriatrics permits a greater diversity of method and emphasis than any other hospital specialty. The authors accept responsibility for the views expressed in this book, but realize that they will not necessarily be shared by all their readers!

Chapter 1
Geriatric Medicine

Geriatric medicine (geriatrics) is that branch of general medicine concerned with the clinical, preventive, remedial and social aspects of illness in elderly people. Their high morbidity rates, different patterns of disease presentation, slower response to treatment and requirements for social support call for special medical skills.

Aims

1 To enable elderly people to lead full and active lives.
2 To prevent, detect early and appropriately treat disease.
3 To mitigate suffering, due to disability and disease and so minimize pre-death dependence.
4 To provide sympathetic medical care and social support in the terminal illness.

Preventive geriatrics

Essentially a primary-care activity involving especially the:
    General practitioner (GP)
    Practice or District (community) nurse
    Health visitor
    Social worker
Achieved by:
    Health education
    Use of available social benefits (financial help and services)
    Early recognition and treatment of disease and disability
This anticipatory care goes well beyond the traditional style of general practice where the GP is activated by the patient. Screening for pre-symptomatic disease in the elderly has been found not to be cost-effective. Case finding, looking for established disease and social disadvantage, is of value (see also Chapter 3).

1

Case finding

1 Target on the over 70s or over 75s, especially those who have:
Recently moved house
Recently discharged from hospital
Been bereaved, divorced, separated

2 Most case finding can be 'opportunist' and as an extension to the ordinary consultation:
Seek problems beyond the present complaint
Evaluate medical diagnosis, functional capacity and
social state

3 Those not seen in consultation are contacted and seen by a doctor, practice nurse or health visitor. A structured questionnaire and simple clinical appraisal is required.

4 A postal survey can be useful to identify old people in need of help.

5 Non-responders/non-attenders should be followed up.

Roles of the geriatrician

1 Ultimate responsibility for inpatients under his care.

2 Leader of the hospital geriatric team to:
Establish and argue case for resources
Decide geriatric operational policies
Orchestrate work of the department
Promote a high standard of medicine in the elderly
Provide clinical management of long-term hospital care

3 Advisor to and liaison with hospital specialties:
Orthopaedics and other surgical specialties
Accident and emergency
General medicine
Psychogeriatrics

4 Advisor to general practitioners:
Telephone consultations
Clinic referrals
Domiciliary consultations

5 Advisor to community services:
Social services
Voluntary bodies, e.g. Age Concern, Help the Aged
Private care agencies

6 Teaching and research.

Organization and operational policies
of the geriatric department

The organization varies with available facilities and the special interests of the clinicians. There is a general agreement in Britain that all the acute assessment wards, the main geriatric outpatient clinics and much of the provision for rehabilitation, should be in the District General Hospital (DGH). This ensures ready access to the full range of diagnostic and treatment facilities as well as good levels of staffing in the different disciplines. In rural areas especially, much of the provision for slower-stream rehabilitation, extended care and day hospital care is located in smaller, more homely hospitals away from the DGH. Ideally this type of provision would be in the community hospitals nearer to the patients' homes.

Styles of practice

There is an important functional relationship between general and geriatric medicine, especially in the acute services with four main styles of practice in the UK.

1 Age-related (separated)
All emergencies above a certain age (other than those where the GP makes prior arrangement with an appropriate consultant) are admitted to separate geriatric wards.

2 Age-related (integrated)
As above but with the acute wards shared by both general and geriatric physicians.

3 Problem-related (separated or integrated)
The acute admissions are selected by nature of illness and social disadvantage rather than merely by age.

4 Fully integrated
General and geriatric physicians share all the acute admissions of all ages.

**Operational policies of the
geriatric department**

1 Acute assessment wards
Patients needing facilities only available at DGH
Some short duration terminal care
Average stay 2–3 weeks

2 Rehabilitation wards
Extended remedial therapy following acute episode
Average stay, weeks or months

3 Extended care wards (longstay)
Terminal care of indefinite duration, i.e. 'permanent home'
Relatives' respite or 'holiday' admissions of high-dependency
patients
Awaiting placement in non-hospital accommodation
Average stay, months or years

4 Outpatient clinics
Referrals from GP and hospital specialties
Emphasis on 'new' cases; follow up best left to GP
Urgent referrals seen within 24 hours

5 Day hospital (see Table 1.3)
Referrals for initial multidisciplinary assessment
Rehabilitation and maintenance, and especially for severely
disabled, relatives' respite

The 'critical' age level is determined by the allocation of resources
and the interests of the consultants. It is necessary for the general
practitioners to be familiar with the local arrangements so that they
may collaborate effectively.

In the UK, most of the work is separate from general medicine
and the three common types of organization are:
1 Acute and rehabilitation in one group of wards and separate
longstay wards.
2 Separate wards for acute, rehabilitation and longstay.
3 All functions (acute, rehabilitation, longstay) in all wards.

The first type tends to have the highest bed-population ratio, the second has the highest throughput and the third has the highest consultant-to-bed ratio.

Admissions

Most cases admitted to the acute wards are medical emergencies, a few are cases for investigation, some are admitted inappropriately when the main problem is social rather than medical. This confers no real benefit on the patient and may make her problems more difficult to resolve. Often a new treatable problem precipitates admission and the long-standing intractable problems prevent discharge.

In general the sooner the patient is admitted after the start of illness, the shorter the hospital stay and the greater the likelihood of returning home.

The main reasons for accepting elderly people for admission are indicated in Table 1.1 and the main reasons for avoiding admission are given in Table 1.2. It is vitally important for all those involved with the care of elderly people to understand the need for proper use of resources.

Table 1.1. Reasons for admitting elderly people to hospital

1 Urgent access to surgical or medical treatment:
   Acute abdomen
   Fracture of femur
   Diabetic coma or pre-coma
   Life-threatening cardiac arrhythmia, acute left ventricular failure
2 To make a diagnosis—patient too ill for outpatient investigation
3 'Therapeutic optimism':
   Refractory heart failure
   Investigation and treatment of severe anaemia
   Recently 'Gone off feet'; for mobilization
4 Access to nursing support:
   When diagnosis is clear but home care is impracticable; stroke, congestive heart failure
   Relatives' respite or 'holiday relief'; when home care is temporarily in abeyance
   Terminal care: often temporary while symptoms relieved or relatives 'recharge batteries'
   Long-term or extended care; where no satisfactory alternative exists

Table 1.2. Reasons for avoiding admission of elderly people to hospital

---

1   Patient unlikely to benefit:
    Diagnosis obvious
    Manageable at home
    Treatment within scope of GP
2   Hospitals are dangerous places:
    Risk of 'hospital' infections and adverse drug reactions
    Worsening of mental confusion
    Dangers of bed rest, pressure sores and falls
    Institutionalization, loss of free choice leads to apathy—a sort of 'mental pressure sore'
3   Loss of ecological niche:
    Loss of network of home supports. Relatives' time and patients' accommodation redeployed
    Deterioration of unoccupied property, destruction of pets
4   More appropriate care is indicated
    Residential care home
    Sheltered housing with increased home support
    Psychiatric ward rather than geriatric ward. Policy of 'any port in a storm' is bad practice; worse for patient and a misuse of resource
5   Rationing resources

Discharges

To meet the ever increasing demand for acute hospital care there is great pressure to discharge patients early. However, the discharge of elderly people should be planned in a thorough way well ahead of the discharge date. This gives the best chance of securing the most appropriate available after-care. It should be explained to the patient and her relatives what is to be arranged and why. When social deprivation and handicap are severe a prior 'home visit' by patient and care practitioner (usually one of the remedial therapists) is made to confirm that the proposed discharge is realistic.

Discharge arrangements: check list
1 Pre-discharge ADL (activities of daily living) assessment? Home visit?
2 GP notified?
3 Can patient cope unaided? If not, is sufficient informal help available?
4 Relatives informed?

5 Domiciliary support services required?
6 Prescribed medication? Is help needed with administration? Provide clear typescript of drug schedule.
7 Attendance at day hospital or day centre?
8 Medical follow up usually by GP; hospital for selected purposes.
9 Transport; for discharge and follow-up.

Rehabilitation
Major disabilities requiring rehabilitation:
    Stroke
    Fractured neck of femur
    Arthritis
    Loss of competence and confidence following acute illness or trauma; especially if pre-existing disability
Length of stay varies with:
    Complexity and severity of illness
    Selected cases admitted direct from home to rehabilitation wards have a much shorter stay in hospital than those transferred from acute beds (see Chapter 6).

Extended, continuing or longstay care

Continuing care is an essential feature of medical practice because some patients have persistent, progressive illness and increasing disability. The majority of those with high dependency are manageable at home when the supporting network is robust but a minority require institutional support of greater or lesser degree, intermittently or long term. A homely, secure environment is required with opportunities for privacy and quiet as well as for bustle, noise and social activity. An abundant participation by relatives, friends and voluntary workers has a humanizing influence. Brain damage and mental disorder loom large in extended care.

Continuing care is expensive on a cost-per-case basis and in the UK its control is one of the geriatrician's prime tasks. He will transfer no patient to this facility until every possible avenue of discharge has been explored and found wanting. He makes regular 'trawls' of the extended care wards to ensure that any patient making a late, often unexpected, recovery, or one who is waiting for alternative accommodation, is not overlooked. He is available to advise the attending GP.

Intermittent, relatives' respite admissions

These admissions extend the use of hospital continuing care. If strain on supporting relatives can be relieved at planned, regular intervals, long-term hospital stay may be avoided. Other families manage without regular relief but with the sure knowledge that if they cannot cope or if they wish to go on holiday, admission will be arranged. While the risks of admission are not to be denied (Table 1.2), these arrangements are highly regarded. The Cambridge scheme is managed by the Geriatric Liaison Health Visitor with consultant guidance.

The geriatric day hospital

The geriatric day hospital provides the diagnostic, treatment and care facilities of the hospital without full board and lodging. A midday meal is provided (Table 1.3). It can be a cost-effective alternative to inpatient care and offers a type of care more suited to the needs and preferences of many patients in the post-acute phase of illness. Patients attend, on average, twice weekly so that each

Table 1.3. Geriatric day hospital—operational policies

Planned Attendance	
Once only	Comprehensive functional assessment Technical procedures, e.g. sigmoidoscopy, bone biopsy, change of catheter, bowel clearance prior to radiology
Short-term	Rehabilitation up to 1 month. Wide range of medical and surgical cases from acute wards, already assessed by geriatrician
Medium-term	Rehabilitation 1–3 months; especially patients with stroke, arthritis, Parkinsonism and fractured neck of femur, may require repeated spells of attendance
Extended care	Long-term care of indefinite duration which just allows families to cope, with high dependency patients. Often punctuated by planned relatives' respite admissions. Typically large psychiatric element or fragile home support network

place supports 2.5 attenders. The recommended number of places in each location is 25–30; the average number of attendances per patient is 20.

Geriatric day care is a consultant-led service with important inputs from medicine, nursing and remedial therapy as well as social work and health visiting. It is expensive, labour intensive and not merely a social club. The work focuses on those in need of specialized help to allow home care to continue. The less severely disabled and those with better home support can usually be rehabilitated as outpatients without the full range of day hospital services.

Relationship to other specialties

Care of the elderly is not the monopoly of the geriatricians, most specialties are involved to some extent. The hospital geriatric services are best seen as an essential element in maintaining patients' independence and only in highly selected cases as a source of long-term care. Timely intervention and successful management of acute and transitory disorders can frequently forestall more serious disorders and disability. Outside the hospital the bulk of the health care of the elderly is provided by the general practitioner and the primary care team.

General medicine

Geriatric help will be required with difficult management problems and in the provision of longstay care, when needed. See also 'Styles of practice' earlier on in this chapter.

Orthopaedic and trauma surgery

The geriatrician is available to give pre- and post-operative medical advice, especially for patients with major fractures and multiple ailments such as heart disease, pneumonia and stroke. He gives guidance in rehabilitation and discharge home or provision of extended care. Similar problems of management, but usually less severe, apply to some cases of elective joint replacement. In certain centres the collaborative approach is achieved by working in a combined orthogeriatric unit.

Accident and emergency department (A&E)
1 About a third of all admissions via A&E are elderly.
2 Self-referral is common and usually appropriate with a high proportion of medical emergencies, especially collapses.
3 The geriatric firm 'on take' can be involved in the process of 'triage'.
4 Guidelines for discharge of elderly patients from A&E should be formulated and adhered to (Table 1.4).

Table 1.4. Guidelines for the discharge of elderly patients from the accident and emergency department

1 Inform patient's GP and practice nurse of reason for attendance, treatment given and aftercare required
2 Avoid discharge during night hours unless suitable transport provided and patient accompanied by competent close friend or relative
3 Ascertain mobility and general ability to cope, especially if patient lives alone
4 Involve social worker if main reason for referral is social
5 Duty psychiatrist to see all attempted suicides or parasuicides
6 Request help from on-call geriatrician or psychogeriatrician as appropriate in the more intractable cases
7 Repeated attendances of A&E call for detailed collaborative review of the patient's management by the family doctor, the relevant medical specialist, the patient and her relatives, the social worker and others in the primary care team

Psychogeriatrics
1 Collaboration between geriatrician and psychiatrist is important.
2 The acute psychogeriatric facility should be in the DGH with some 20–30 beds for the average health district.
3 The patients admitted here usually will have multiple illnesses and disabilities.

Resources required

Geriatrics requires considerable hospital facilities as well as backup in the community of a multitude of resources controlled by the local authority, voluntary bodies and private agencies. Table 1.5 gives some indication of the extent of provision in the hospital service. See Chapter 3 for information regarding community services.

Table 1.5. Guidelines for resources: geriatric units in England and Wales

---

Beds:
    10 per 1000 population age 65}; 30–50 per cent in DGH; actual requirement depends upon other local resources

Day hospital places:
    1.5–2.0 places per 1000 population age 65}; 30–40 per cent in DGH

Outpatient clinics:
    Located mostly in the DGH to give ready access to diagnostic facilities

Consultants:
    1 WTE for not more than 70 beds and 20 day hospital places; increments required for geographical spread, involvement in management, teaching, etc

Other medical staff:
    WTE per 24 beds in the DGH:
        1 house officer   all below SR to
        1 senior house officer   rotate with
        ½ registrar or senior registrar   general medicine
    Non-acute beds to have a much reduced level of staffiing; may rely on clinical assistants

Nurses:
    Minimum ratio of 1 nurse to 1.16 patients, most to be trained general nurses. On non-acute wards up to 50 per cent may be less highly trained

Remedial therapists:
    Per 200 beds plus 40 day hospital places
    7 physiotherapists plus 7 helpers
    7 occupational therapists plus 7 helpers
    2 speech therapists

    Additionally there are guidelines for social workers, liaison community nurses, health visitors, dieticians, chiropodists, etc.

WTE = Whole-time equivalents.
(Based on BGS recommendations, 1982)

Geriatrics as a career

Geriatrics, is the third largest of the medical specialties in the UK with over 500 consultants and excellent career prospects for the foreseeable future. The physician in geriatric medicine needs to be an able manager, a team leader as well as a good clinician. Most British medical schools offer some experience and instruction in the subject and geriatrics features as part of the final examination in medicine. An increasing number of able graduates are attracted to a career in the specialty (see Table 1.6).

Table 1.6. Why geriatrics?

Clinical and organizational challenge—one of the biggest and most pressing in medicine

Multidisciplinary working

Continuity of care and community involvement

Can often do very much more to help than the patient expects—cure occasionally, ameliorate often, helpful always

Scope for innovative practice and research

Career opportunities in an international health growth area

Training in geriatrics

A career in geriatrics requires at least 3 years' grounding in general professional work at senior house officer and registrar level. Mostly this would be in general medicine but some time in related specialties such as geriatrics, neurology, psychiatry, rheumatology or general practice would be useful. During general professional training the doctor should secure Membership of the Royal College of Physicians (UK).

Higher specialist training at senior registrar (SR) level may be solely in geriatrics or in combined general medicine and geriatrics. Those interested in an academic career might do well to take a research post (from 1–3 years) leading to a PhD or MD. At least 2 years must be spent in an accredited post in geriatrics at SR level but experience in related specialties is encouraged. After appropriate training the doctor is eligible to apply for appointment as:

1 Consultant in geriatric medicine.

2 Consultant in general medicine, with a special interest in the elderly.

3 Senior lecturer/consultant in an academic department with a view to possible professorship or eventual return to non-academic NHS work.

For doctors with special domestic commitments, disability or ill health, part-time training is possible but takes more years to complete. Further information on geriatrics as a career is obtainable from the nearest medical school or the British Geriatrics Society, 1 St Andrews Place, Regents Park, London NW1 4LE.

Further reading

Andrews K. & Brocklehurst J.C. (1985) Profile of geriatric rehabilitation units. *Journal of the Royal College of Physicians*, **19**, 240–2.

British Geriatrics Society (1986) *Guidelines for Provision of Adequate Services in Geriatric Medicine*. London.

Brocklehurst J.C. (1985) The geriatric service and the day hospital. In: Brocklehurst J.C. (ed.) *Textbook of Geriatric Medicine and Gerontology*, pp. 982–95. Churchill Livingstone, Edinburgh.

Brocklehurst J.C. & Andrews K. (1985) Geriatric medicine—the style of practice. *Age and Ageing*, **14**, 1–7.

Williams E.I. (1985) Anticipatory care for the elderly in general practice. In: Isaacs B. (ed.) *Recent Advances in Geriatric Medicine*, Vol. 3, pp. 255–63. Churchill Livingstone, Edinburgh.

Chapter 2
Demography of Ageing and Care in the Community

Population trends

These are clearly illustrated in Table 2.1. There are marked differences between the developed and developing countries. The prime reason for the worldwide increase in the proportion of elderly subjects is the combined effect of declining child mortality with a falling birth rate. Consequences and solutions will depend on the levels of economic and educational development within individual countries.

Developed countries

- There has been a dramatic rise in the elderly throughout the present century but this is now slowing down.
- However, the old old, i.e. greater than 80 years of age, are still increasing rapidly.
- A sophisticated medical service is established.
- Specialist services for the elderly are available.
- The rising expectations of the elderly and their supporters and carers will result in rising costs.
- UK population trends alone demand a 1 per cent increase in health funding in addition to inflation costs (approximately 5 per cent) and costs due to technological development.
- Costs may be reduced by health promotion, disease prevention and self-reliance schemes.
- Ethical dilemmas must be addressed, for example, prolongation of death by technological intervention or medicated survival of young chronic sick and acutely ill frail elderly patients.
- Financial consequences of decisions must be calculated and proper provisions made to support the choice made. An elderly

Table 2.1. Population in millions (1980–2000)

	Total population			Population 60+			Population 70+			Population 80+		
	1980	2000	Increase %	1980	2000	Increase %	1980	2000	Increase %	1980	2000	Increase %
Australia	14.5	17.8	23	1.9	2.7	38.7	0.8	1.3	58.7	0.2	0.3	61.4
Brazil	122.3	187.5	53	7.5	14.0	86.7	3.0	6.0	100.0	0.7	1.6	117.1
Egypt	42.0	64.4	53	2.4	4.6	91.7	0.8	1.7	112.5	0.1	0.3	146.9
FRG	60.9	58.8	–3	11.4	13.3	16.9	6.0	6.1	1.1	1.5	1.7	12.8
France	53.5	56.3	5	9.1	10.8	19.4	5.1	5.6	10.4	1.4	1.5	4.9
India	684.5	960.6	40	33.9	65.7	93.8	11.1	22.4	101.8	2.0	3.6	80.0
Israel	3.9	5.6	44	0.4	0.6	38.2	0.2	0.3	50.0	0.04	0.08	100.0
Italy	56.9	59.1	4	10.0	13.5	34.6	5.0	6.9	38.0	1.2	1.9	55.5
Japan	116.6	129.3	11	14.8	26.4	78.4	6.4	11.9	85.9	1.5	3.0	102.5
Kenya	16.5	30.4	84	0.7	1.3	85.7	0.3	0.5	6.7	0.04	0.1	150.0
Nigeria	77.1	150.0	95	3.1	6.4	106.5	1.0	2.2	120.0	0.2	0.4	155.3
Philippines	49.2	77.0	57	2.2	4.6	109.1	0.7	1.7	142.9	0.1	0.3	114.5
Poland	35.8	41.2	15	4.7	6.8	44.7	2.3	3.2	39.1	0.5	0.7	50.0
Sweden	8.3	8.1	–2	1.8	1.8	–1.8	0.9	1.0	11.1	0.2	0.3	36.9
United Kingdom	55.9	55.2	–1	11.1	11.3	1.3	5.4	6.0	11.1	1.4	1.8	28.6
USA	223.2	263.8	18	33.9	40.1	18.3	H5.6	20.6	32.1	4.4	5.8	31.8
World	4432.1	6118.8	38	375.8	590.4	57.1	158.3	252.3	59.5	35.3	59.6	68.8

(Source: Provisional projections of the United Nations Population Division, New York, 1980)

person costs the health service nine times as much as a young subscriber.

1980/81 UK health costs per head (age 16–64) £85

1980/81 UK health costs per head (age 75+) £765

Developing countries

• These countries are about to experience a massive and rapid distortion of previous population patterns.

• Rising number of elderly people will coincide with falling birth rate, as contraceptive policies become effective.

• Their health services are often primitive, patchy and inappropriate to needs.

• There are many other pressing financial demands for expansion, e.g. education, housing and development of infrastructure.

• Economic dependence on developed countries is restrictive.

• Political instability is common.

• Social structure likely to be rapidly altered, e.g. by population migration.

• Potentially preventable disabilities acquired in youth will complicate old age.

• The poor will be unable to acquire sufficient wealth to provide for themselves in old age, therefore the total burden will fall on provision by the state or the problem will be neglected.

Where do the elderly live in the United Kingdom

In the 'community'—96 per cent

In institutions—4 per cent

Housing

• In the United Kingdom the largest housing category is owner occupiers and accounts for about 50 per cent.

• A high percentage of elderly people (compared with the young) are in rented accommodation—about one-third in council property and half as many in the private sector.

• Elderly people have a higher share of poor housing; the old tend to live in the oldest housing, almost half of the unfit housing in the UK (e.g. lacking one basic amenity, i.e. inside WC, bath, shower, hot water supply) is occupied by persons over the age of 65 years.

• Five per cent of the elderly population in the United Kingdom live in special accommodation, i.e. purpose built with warden support (sheltered housing).

Sheltered accommodation
This, in the main, is characterized by:
• Purpose built (bungalows or flats which are served by a resident warden).
• Based on the almshouse principle but rapidly expanded in the 1960s and 70s.
• Mainly built by local authorities or housing associations.
• Tenants rarely move, therefore old schemes have very old and frail occupants—causing much stress and strain on the warden.
• Schemes attractive to active elderly couples also need to be suitable for disabled and solitary occupation.
• Residents often make heavy demands on supporting services—the warden alone is rarely sufficient and officially only available to summon help when required. Many wardens often do much more. Demands on isolated wardens have not been matched by increased levels of training, relief arrangements or by remuneration. There is therefore much discontent and anxiety.
• Elderly people are often encouraged to apply for sheltered accommodation by their relatives who feel that their responsibilities and obligations have then been fulfilled. However, informal carer support should still be an important ingredient to life in sheltered accommodation.

Very sheltered accommodation
This is purpose built for the very frail elderly and includes provision for extra staffing levels. These schemes have developed because of the success of sheltered housing, making it possible to keep elderly people in the community and because of the failure of residential care to provide sufficient or attractive accommodation for the increasingly dependent.

Very sheltered accommodation is usually attached to a standard sheltered accommodation complex. Such schemes require a major input from other local authority and NHS supporting services.

'Stayput' schemes
These are to enable elderly people to stay in their familiar environment by improving the safety and convenience of their own

home. There are considerable advantages in staying in a familiar environment surrounded by familiar neighbours. The support that they can offer may be irreplaceable.

The provision of money and assistance to modify housing according to needs dictated by disability is an essential requirement for 'stayput' schemes.

The development of alarm systems which can be easily and cheaply installed and served by peripatetic wardens also facilitates the development of 'stayput' schemes.

Community care in the United Kingdom

Currently fashionable for the elderly, the mentally ill and mentally and physically handicapped of all ages. Most elderly people wish to continue to live in their own home but the cost-effectiveness of this is dubious when considerable statutory support is required. There is also a high social cost to the informal carers.

Forty-five per cent of elderly women and 17 per cent of elderly men live alone—the percentage rises for both sexes with increasing age. In all, one-third of pensioners live alone; half of them live with their spouses and only one-fifth live with their family (children or siblings) or friends. The multiple generation (extended family) is rare in the United Kingdom and has probably always been so.

Who cares?

Informal carers
These are the most important members of the caring workforce. They are unpaid, untrained, but devoted and effective. Although the generations tend to live apart there continues to be frequent contact within a family and almost 50 per cent of elderly people living alone have regular daily contact with a family member. The bulk of community support is provided by family and friends—the following points are relevant to the situation within the United Kingdom:

• The proportion of dependents, i.e. children under 16, men over 65 and women over 60 in the community, has not increased during this century (see Table 2.2).

• There are now more dependent elderly people in the community than dependent children.

Table 2.2. Percentage of dependents in the community, i.e. pensioners and children

Year	%
1901	41
1951	37
1981	40
1991	39
2001	40

• It is calculated that in the United Kingdom 1.25 million people care for elderly dependents.

• Most carers are women (60 per cent) and over half of 'housewives' can expect to be called upon at some time to help an elderly and infirm person. Thirteen per cent of all women have current caring responsibilities to old people and this rises to 20 per cent in women over the age of 40 years.

• Many carers are themselves pensioners. The mean age of carers of confused elderly people is 61 years.

Statutory services

The so-called statutory services are provided in combination by the local authority, which is financed through the general rates and NHS staff who are funded by central government. Sometimes the local authority services are delegated to voluntary organizations who act as agents. Services may be obtained by application to the Departments of Social Services or through the Primary Health Care Team. They may be free or a token charge may be made. This will depend on the local arrangements within the local authority. NHS services are mostly provided free of charge and are arranged through the patient's registered general practitioner. Where NHS charges do exist, there is usually exemption for people of pensionable age or financial assistance can be obtained.

Local authority services

Home-help service

This is the lynchpin of organized community support. It initially started as a domestic service with the provision of help with cleaning but has gradually expanded to cover cooking, shopping and personal attention. Because of its expanded role it is now sometimes described as a domiciliary care service. There is no recognized training scheme for home-helps/domiciliary care assistants but local training schemes are now being organized.

Visits by the service may range from a few hours per week up to 3 or more visits a day depending on the client's needs and availability of the service. A good home-help is priceless and can give immeasurable help and assistance to very frail elderly people who, without such care, would be non-viable within the community. Because of the great individual variation found in home-helps and in clients, a great deal of skill is needed by the Home-Help Coordinator to ensure a perfect match between helper and client.

Although an expanding service the number of home-helps has not kept up with demographic trends (see Table 2.3).

Table 2.3. Home-help provision in the UK

	1975–76	1981–82
Home-help whole-time equivalent per thousand population	50	51
Per thousand population over 75 years	20.5	18

Meals-on-wheels service

This provides clients with hot meals in their own home, usually for a nominal charge. Initiated mainly by voluntary organizations (especially the Women's Royal Voluntary Service) it has been gradually taken over by Departments of Social Services.
- Meals are provided daily (at mid-day) but usually just 2 or 3 times per week.
- Provision of the service is patchy and in many areas, especially rural ones, it is impossible to provide weekend meals.
- There are great practical problems in providing meals which remain appetizing and nutritious after delays caused by preparation, storage and delivery.
- Alternative methods of providing a regular meal service have been tried, e.g. frozen meals which require reheating and boil-in-

the-bag prepared meals. Many in need are too disabled to cope with such systems.

• If mainly dependent on meals-on-wheels for nutrition more than 4 meals per week are required to fulfill the recommended minimal dietary requirements.

• Currently in the UK more than 26 million meals are provided by this service each year and about 3 per cent of elderly people benefit, rising to 12 per cent in the over 85s.

• This service would be more efficient if there was improved supervision as some meals are inappropriate.

• There is little social benefit from eating alone. See Table 2.4 for advantages and disadvantages of meals-on-wheels.

Table 2.4. Reasons for meals-on-wheels

Good reasons	Poor reasons
1 To relieve other carers who normally provide meals	1 Being housebound, where a shopping service is needed, i.e. client can cook but has mobility problems which prevent shopping
2 Where severe irreversible physical disability prevents cooking or makes it unacceptably dangerous	2 Social isolation where apathy or depression interfere with nutrition—these people will attain greater benefit from attendance at a luncheon club or day centre
3 Where severe intellectual failure interferes with meal planning and preparation	3 Uncompensated disability where clients could cook if advised by an occupational therapist about necessary aids which would be provided to overcome this disability
4 As a temporary measure whilst recovering from a reversible condition which is being treated	4 Unrecognized and untreated medical conditions where a correctable medical problem interferes with the patient's ability to cope, for example, congestive heart failure and cataracts
	5 Poverty—provision of additional funds will allow client to cook and to exercise choice
	6 Ignorance about dietary requirements—education should be provided

Luncheon clubs

These are centres where meals are provided, usually at subsidized prices, run either by the local authority or voluntary organizations. They provide meals to 3 per cent of the elderly population, i.e. similar provision to meals-on-wheels service. Frequency of meal provision from luncheon clubs is less than that provided by the meals-on-wheels service—usually just once or twice weekly but companionship is offered in addition to food.

There are often problems concerning access to luncheon clubs, i.e. many attenders need to have transport provided which considerably increases costs. Attendance gives the opportunity to disseminate health education and other relevant information concerning support services.

Day centres

These are very varied and may be run by the local authority or voluntary groups and must not be confused with day hospitals. They may be housed in purpose-built accommodation, modified buildings or multi-purpose community halls, etc. They may be freestanding or attached to another institution, e.g. local authority residential care homes or school buildings. Staff may be trained (social workers, therapists) or untrained or a combination of both. A charge for attendance is usually made and transport may be provided. About 5 per cent of elderly people attend day centres. The aims of the day centres are:

>   To combat loneliness
>   To provide diversional activity and recreation
>   To provide a meal and other comforts
>   To relieve other supporters
>   To introduce clients to other forms of care
>   To disseminate health education, etc.

National Health Service community services

General practitioners

In the UK every person is registered with a general practitioner who acts as the first point of contact for all NHS services. If multidisciplinary care is to succeed in the community setting it is essential that the general practitioner becomes the effective leader of the

team. The good general practitioner needs:
- A wide knowledge of both medicine and the scope of the skills and abilities of the other team members.
- Comprehensive records detailing the patient's past medical history.
- Up-to-date information about patient's current problems and treatment.
- A friendly and approachable manner so that neither elderly patients or their carers (formal or informal) are deterred from seeking his help.
- A regular review of the elderly, sick and the vulnerable in his practice.
- Ready access to specialists' (hospital-based) help and advice.

Table 2.5. Community services received by 265 dependent people over 70 years of age and living in their own homes in Wales

Services	%
Informal carers	89
Home-helps	17
Meals-on-wheels	7
Social workers	5
Nurses	20
Day Hospitals	11
Occupational therapists	1
Physiotherapists	1
Volunteers	2

NB   Only 28 out of 265 relied entirely on statutory services

In England and Wales there are almost 26000 general practitioners. On average each of them has 400 people of pensionable age on their lists. However, there is wide geographical variation and some general practitioners have a much higher proportion of elderly patients—sometimes by choice—especially if he is a member of a group practice and has had a special interest and training in the problems of the elderly.

Anticipatory care in the community
In general practice in the United Kingdom there are many potential opportunities for doctors to prevent illness and encourage

improved health in elderly people. An age/sex register is essential for such activities.

Health education (primary prevention)
1 Knowledge about ageing and age-related illness should be disseminated to all age-groups throughout life.
2 Retirement courses with contributions from the entire Primary Health Care Team should be arranged by group practices. Such activity will both instruct the elderly in how to avoid or prevent disease in old age and facilitate relationships between potential patients and medical and other staff.

Potentially preventable diseases in old age
1 Multi-infarct dementia and stroke by treatment of blood pressure.
2 Osteoporosis by hormone-replacement therapy in post-menopausal women.
3 Ischaemic heart disease by dietary change and avoidance of tobacco.
4 Alcoholic dementia, heart failure, pancreatitis and cirrhosis.
5 Obesity and its effect on osteoarthritis and carbohydrate metabolism.
6 Diverticular disease and gall bladder disease by attention to dietary fibre.
7 Chronic obstructive airways disease and bronchogenic carcinoma, risks reduced by tobacco abstinence.
8 Dietary deficiency states.
9 Iatrogenic disease.

Screening programmes (secondary prevention)
Ideally involves the examination and investigation of all elderly people within a population:
    Identifies undetected and asymptomatic disease
    Expensive in time, money and manpower
    Considered obtrusive by some patients
    Not all detected pathology will be treatable
    Compliance with treatment in asymptomatic disease is poor in elderly patients
    Generally, blanket-screening or visiting is not considered to be

cost-effective. Routine examination of peripheral blood-films and urine examination are considered the most valuable activities. Work can be delegated to nurses and other members of the multi-disciplinary team.

Case finding (tertiary prevention)
This is where patients with an established disease and disability are sought and early intervention instigated in order to limit the consequences of the problems:
- Postal surveys can be used to identify patients in difficulty.
- Efforts can be concentrated on at risk groups, for example:
    The very old (over 80 years)
    The recently bereaved or separated
    The socially isolated
    The poor
    The recently moved (change-of-dwelling)
    The recently ill
- Cases worth finding, for example:
    Those with failing vision and hearing
    Patients with mobility problems
    Patients with difficulty in self-care
    Patients with reduced effort tolerance
    Patients with falling weight
    The depressed
    Non-responders to questionnaires

Opportunistic case finding
During any consultation the opportunity should be taken to enquire about other health or social problems. Well elderly clinics are for the worried-well and for those not sure about their health or abilities.

Community nursing staff

Community sisters—district nurses
Eighty per cent of the total time of these nurses is devoted to the care of elderly people, they provide:
    Hands-on-nursing
    Treatment, e.g. injections, enemas and dressings

Specialist care, e.g. stoma management and continence advice
Liaison with other services

Health visitors
Only 15 per cent of their time is devoted to the care of the elderly
and, at present, their involvement with this age group appears to be
declining. However, they play a valuable role with regard to the
following:
Advise, counsel and educate
Identify needs
Practise prevention
Liaise with other services

Community psychiatric nurses
This is a small but expanding group of community workers and their
main tasks are:
To support the patients and carers
To monitor progress or deterioration
To liaise with other services
NB   All community nurses require specialist training in
community needs and techniques. The nursing staff may be
augmented by less specialized aides and informal carers.

Institutional care
This is available and necessary for only a minority of elderly people
(4 per cent in the UK) and is unlikely to expand rapidly. The
proportion of elderly people in care is much higher in other
European and Western countries than in the UK. See Tables 2.6
and 2.7 for provision in England and Wales.

Reasons for institutionalization
• Severe physical disabilities.
• Immobile without help.
• Severe mental disabilities, constant supervision needed.
• Passive/dependent personality.
• Hostile community or non-existent community support.
• Wealth makes choice possible between community and insti-
tutional care.
NB   Usually at least two criteria are required in the UK to qualify
for care.

Table 2.6. Non-psychiatric institutional beds for the elderly (England 1984)

NHS geriatric beds in hospitals	53 000 (19% of total)
Private nursing homes	28 000 (10% of total)
Local authority residential care	110 000 (39% of total)
Private residential homes	90 000 (32% of total)
Total	280 000

Table 2.7. Hospital inpatient enquiry—occupancy by age of hospital beds excluding maternity and psychiatry 1981

	All ages	%65–74	%75–84	%85 }	%over 65 years
All specialties	161 372	20.5	26.4	13.3	60.2
General medicine	25 354	28.4	20.9	6.5	55.8
General surgery	21 770	24.6	18.3	4.2	47.1
Orthopaedic surgery	16 780	17.1	20.6	11.0	48.7
Geriatric beds	51 306	20.0	46.4	29.4	95.8

Table 2.8. Characteristics of residents

A census undertaken in January 1983 of 1246 residents of the 32 old people's homes in Cambridgeshire showed:

    71.6% are women
    over two-thirds of residents are over 80
    18.5% of residents are over 90
    Few are blind, but 20.1% are partially sighted
    25.2% are hard of hearing
    4.3% are profoundly deaf
    Almost half use walking aids, only 10% of residents can walk with very little help
    21.3% require help with toileting
    13.6% are incontinent of urine at night
    11.4% are incontinent of urine by day
    13.2% are severely confused
    32.8% are mildly confused and 4.1% are mentally handicapped
    56.8% come from within a 5-mile radius of the home, and a further 20.4% come from 5–10 miles away
    84.7% of residents never go out alone, but 17.1% go out regularly, if accompanied
    47.2% watch TV regularly
    56.2% have visits from family/relatives regularly

Complications of institutionalization
- Depersonalization.
- Marked restriction of choices.
- Accelerated dependence.

NB   All of these can be avoided by persistent effort by residents and staff.

Residential care

In the UK this is provided by both the local authority and the private sector—but there is no uniformity of geographical availability.

Most residents on entry are now over 80 years of age and suffer from multiple disabilities (both physical and mental, see Table 2.8).

Medical cover is provided by the resident's own general practitioner and if nursing help is required for specific tasks, this is provided by the community nursing staff as if the patient was still living in her own home. The permanent staff of the home will be either residential social workers or care assistants—other specialist help may be available on demand from the usual domiciliary services.

Further reading

Hobman D. (ed.) (1981) *The Impact of Ageing.* Croom Helm, London.
Kinmaid J., Batherston J. & Williamson J. (eds) (1981) *The Provision of Care for the Elderly.* Churchill Livingstone, Edinburgh.
Selby P. & Schechter M. (eds) (1982) *Ageing 2000—a Challenge for Society.* MTP Press, Lancaster.
Tinker A. (1984) *The Elderly in Modern Society.* Longman, Essex.

Chapter 3
Social Aspects of Ageing

Old age is unfortunately often a time of loss. The potential losses are very varied but are often inter-related and the ones that accompany old age are:
- Health due to increasing pathology.
- Wealth due to termination of employment.
- Companionship secondary to bereavement.
- Independence due to acquired disabilities.
- Homeostasis due to loss of fine control over internal environment.
- Status following retirement and loss of independence.

The above changes and losses may expose the elderly person to the following consequences:
- Unhappiness, grief, depression, suicide (see Chapters 7 & 21).
- Increased incidence of illness.
- Increased risk of accident.
- Poverty.
- Dependence and abuse.
- Malnutrition and subnutrition.
- Hypothermia (see Chapter 15).
- Retirement.

Loss of wealth

Income falls on the giving-up of paid employment. Pensions are not normally equivalent to wages and on average the pension is approximately 50 per cent of the average working wage for a couple (see Table 3.1). Increasing frailty may seriously restrict choice and lead to loss of opportunities to economize. Disabilities themselves may result in additional costs, e.g. for help, aids and adaptations.

The elderly spend a much higher percentage of their total expenditure on essentials, e.g. heating, food, housing and the opportunity to economize is not common. The safety net provided

Table 3.1. Pensions as percentage of average earnings in manufacturing 1975 (for an aged couple)

Austria	54
Canada	57
Denmark	43
France	65
FRG	50
Italy	67
Netherlands	54
Norway	55
Sweden	76
Switzerland	53
UK	39
USA	57

(Source: *Social Security Bulletin*, Jan. 1978)

by the social security system is complex and difficult and this alone acts as a deterrent to the taking-up of additional benefits. This system is always changing in an attempt to cut costs.

Allowances which can be claimed by some UK pensioners

1 Supplementary pension—savings must be less than £3000. Value of home not included, but any other properties must be taken into account. Possible additions are available for:

Age over 80
Blindness
Mortgage interest
Water rates
Ground rent and service charges
House insurance
Special diets
Special laundry, e.g. for incontinence
Heating
Hospital fares and other special transport costs
Board and lodging for residential care and nursing homes

2 Single payments—payable when savings are less than £500 for replacement of clothing, repairs to home, redecoration, bedding and furniture.

3 Housing benefit from the local Authority Housing Department for rent or rates.

4 Attendance allowance (day or night allowances)—only paid for disabilities of greater duration than 6 months.

5 Mobility allowance may be carried over for 10 years after 65 years, if claimed before that time.

6 Death grant to help pay for funerals and if extra financial help is required, it must be requested before the funeral is carried out.

7 Extra money for carers:

(i) Invalid care allowance for a carer who earns less than £12 per week and who provides more than 35 hours of care per week.

(ii) Home responsibility protection to protect pension rights of carers.

NB For current details see Age Concern Publication, *Your Rights.*

Subnutrition

In the UK subnutrition is rarely due to poverty. It is more likely to be a consequence of eccentricity, illness or loneliness. Overnutrition with excess of carbohydrate, fat and calories is of greater frequency than malnutrition and these excesses are often associated with a deficient amount of dietary fibre. Displacement of nutrients by alcohol abuse is another significant cause for dietary distortion. Other important factors related to diet in old age are as follows:

• The incidence of subnutrition is difficult to determine as dietary assessment by recall (of foods eaten) or weighed surveys are unreliable in many elderly subjects and particularly in the most vulnerable.

• There is considerable doubt about the accuracy of recommended intakes—in elderly may need more or less than some other groups.

• United Kingdom surveys in the 1960s and 70s indicated levels of malnutrition of about 3–7 per cent.

• Poor diets may be either the result or the cause of declining health.

• Other factors are social isolation and bereavement.

• Low blood levels of vitamins, etc. are common in old age, especially in the frail elderly, but their significance is uncertain (see Table 3.2).

Causes of nutritional deficiency

1 Inability to shop or to prepare food, e.g. in cases of dementia,

Table 3.2. Incidence of low blood levels of vitamins, etc. that have been reported in elderly subjects

Haemoglobin less than 12 g	up to 40% in institutions
	6–9% elderly at home
Serum iron	approx 20%
Red cell folate	approx 20%
Serum B_{12}	approx 20%
Red cell B_6	approx 6%
Vitamin C	up to 50%
Vitamin D	up to 70%

NB   Wide variation due to different groups studied and methods used—all incidences of low levels are more common than actual evidence of clinical deficiences.

depression, blindness or immobility due to arthritis or neurological disease.

2 Impaired appetite which may be part of the clinical picture of general malaise, may be due to biochemical abnormalities, a consequence of the side effects of drugs, or may indicate underlying gastrointestinal disease.

3 Malabsorption (see Chapter 14).

A simple recipe for a good diet
1 Eat wholemeal bread, not white bread.
2 Have two portions of fresh vegetables daily.
3 Eat one item of fresh fruit each day.
4 Use 1 pint of skimmed milk daily, for drinking and for use as an ingredient in cooking.
5 Have 1 egg per day.
6 Have 1 portion of meat or fish per day.
7 Drink at least 2 litres of fluid a day.

Assessment of nutritional status in old age
This is a very difficult task but the following criteria have been found to be of value:
• Dietary history.
• Weight change.
• Height change.
• Skinfold thickness.
• Muscle power.

- Blood levels of nutrients.
- Clinical evidence of nutritional disease.

Taken in isolation most of these abnormalities have multiple causes. A diagnosis of malnutrition can only be made if several abnormalities are found—the cause of the malnutrition must then be explored and, if possible, corrected.

Dietary deficiencies in old age

1 Vitamin B group—refractory heart failure, macrocytic anaemia due to folate deficiency, also peripheral neuropathy and dementia.
2 Vitamin C—scurvy.
3 Vitamin D—osteomalacia.
4 Fibre—diseases of 'Western civilization'.

Treatment of subnutrition

1 Improve general health—treat underlying conditions.
2 Supplement intake—meals-on-wheels, luncheon clubs, meal preparation by home-help, give vitamin supplements
(see Chapter 2).
3 Education of patients and carers.

Old-age abuse

This is both difficult to define and detect. It is not restricted simply to physical violence, such as pushing, punching and slapping but may also take other forms as follows:
- Psychological—shouting and/or blackmail.
- Financial—'asset-stripping'.
- Emotional.
- Neglect—withholding food, drink and warmth.
- Sexual.

American studies indicate that the incidence of old-age abuse may be as high as 10 per cent amongst dependent elderly people. In one survey of carers 40 per cent admitted to screaming and yelling, 6 per cent to physical restraint, 6 per cent to forced feeding and forced medication, 6 per cent threatened abandonment to an institution, 4 per cent threatened physical violence and 3 per cent admitted to continual slapping. Most instances of abuse are a symptom of a carer under stress, e.g. in the following cases:
1 Resentful carer because of marked sudden or unexpected change in lifestyle caused by adoption of caring role.

2 Carer with divided loyalties, e.g. to an elderly parent and to a child (the torn middle generation).

3 Carer with health problems of her own, e.g. alcoholism.

4 Role reversal, e.g. ageing, unmarried child caring for an aged parent.

The elderly at special risk are thought to fall into the following categories:

• The heavily dependent.

• Those with communication problems, e.g. dementia, deafness or impaired comprehension.

• Those in cramped and unsatisfactory housing.

The diagnosis of abuse is often very difficult to make and difficult to substantiate. However, the following warning signs may be of value:

• Recurrent falls and accidents.

• Multiple bruising, especially clear thumb prints inflicted during an episode of shaking, also bruises and burns in unusual places, e.g. flexure surfaces.

• Excessive requests for repeat prescriptions.

• A carer complaining of 'nerves' or a carer under stress (see previous list).

Bereavement
See Chapter 21.

Retirement

Compulsory retirement has distorted ageing in Western society. In underdeveloped countries elderly people are able to continue with physical labour until overcome by illness—they do not lose muscle bulk and strength to the same degree as their Western counterparts.

In the West many self-employed people continue to work well beyond the age of retirement, e.g. general practitioners, politicians, writers, actors and painters.

Compulsory retirement is used to control the balance between employment and unemployment rates in industrial society—but this is not necessarily in the best interests of the individual. Retirement is a mixed blessing. Twenty per cent of workers fear retirement but 50 per cent look forward to it. The negative aspects of retirement are as follows:

- Loss of income, everybody becomes poorer.
- Loss of status associated with work.
- Loss of companionship from workmates.
- Loss of health.
- Realization of mortality.

To counteract the above disadvantages, there are the following positive aspects of retirement:

- It may occupy one-third of your life.
- You may remain fit and healthy for most of this time.
- It is an opportunity to redesign your life and to promote good health.
- Time is available for new interests, activities and relationships.

Retirement may bring social problems of its own and it is a time when some difficult decisions will have to be made. Dilemmas encountered may include the following:

- Becoming a carer, e.g. of your parents at the beginning of retirement or your spouse or siblings at the end of retirement.
- Where to live—probably best to stay where you are comfortable and are well known. If a move is contemplated then earlier is better than later when you will be fitter and more likely to be one of a pair.
- What sort of accommodation?—somewhere where you are able to be independent, even in spite of acquired disabilities.
- Driving—you may need to give up at some stage—so beware of geographical isolation (see Chapter 8).
- Sex—'it is allowed' even in very old age so long as it gives pleasure to all concerned (see Chapter 16).
- Boredom affects 10 per cent of the retired—another 20 per cent (although not bored) would prefer still to be working. The poor, the disabled and poorly educated and the isolated are most likely to be dissatisfied with retirement.

Preparation for retirement

This should be lifelong (remember that the poorly educated fare badly after retirement). Attendance at pre-retirement courses should be encouraged, but they often provide too little too late and only reach the well-motivated. Nevertheless, they are useful and provide an opportunity to disseminate positive aspects about retirement. However, the more negative aspects of retirement should not be overlooked although the participants in the course may be reluctant to consider these. In general pre-retirement courses provide an opportunity to give health education and information to a captive audience.

Health topics for retirement lectures

1 Positive health
Diet—low fat, high fibre, calorie control.
Physical exercise—must be graduated, regular and enjoyable.
Mental exercise—encourage the development of new skills and knowledge.
Avoid harmful habits, e.g. tobacco, alcohol and obesity.

2 Information about health problems
Arthritis and other locomotor problems.
Vascular diseases—including heart disease and stroke.
Impairment of special senses.
Difficulty in bladder and bowel control.

3 Provision of information
About available services, including how and when to obtain them and use them.

4 Breaking taboos
Death and bereavement.
Sex in old age.
Fitness to drive.
Dementia and depression.
Caring for dependent relatives.

Further reading

Armstrong J., Midwinter G. & Wynne-Horley D. (1987) *Retired Leisure*. Centre for Policy on Ageing, London.

Kemm J.R. (ed.) (1985) *Vitamin Deficiency in the Elderly*. Blackwell Scientific Publications, Oxford.

Selby P. & Griffiths A. (1986) *A Guide to Successful Ageing*. Parthenon Publishing, London.

Also see reading list for Chapter 2.

Chapter 4
The Ageing Process

One of the great successes of civilization has been the emergence of senescence as a phenomenon affecting mankind, particularly in the European countries but, as we have seen in Chapter 2, increasingly in the developing world as well. Populations of animal species do not exhibit this phenomenon except under artificial conditions, so the biological study of the ageing process is not a simple matter. Nevertheless, a number of observations have contributed to a growing understanding of some of the mechanisms involved, and the more important of these will be summarized.

1 The mathematical model (Gompertz)
Ageing is an increasing probability of death, this probability doubling every 8 years after the age of thirty. Human mortality is at its lowest at the age of 12 in all countries studied. A consignment of glass tumblers in a canteen has been suggested as an example of a population which might not exhibit the characteristics of senescence (see Fig. 4.1) although this is not entirely true, chipped tumblers are at a greater risk of subsequent cracking.

2 An evolutionary adaptation
Death, and therefore an increasing liability to death in a population which has largely conquered random loss through natural disaster, is a social necessity. 'While there's death there's hope.'

3 Loss of non-replicating cells
Neuronal, renal and myocardial cells have to last a lifetime. A steady decline in number occurs, for example, through micro-environmental insults or genetic mechanisms.

4 Production of unsound cells (Orgel)
Self-reproducing errors accumulate in proteins and enzymes faster than they are detected or repaired, eventually damaging

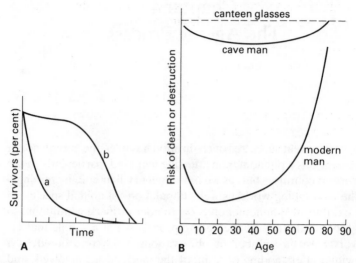

Fig. 4.1. A: Survival curves of populations (a) showing constant rate of mortality of 50 per cent per unit time and (b) showing senescence (Source: Comfort A. [1979]: *The Biology of Senescence*, 3rd ed. Churchill Livingstone, Edinburgh). **B:** Ageing as a risk of death (or destruction) in the two populations (Source: Coni N.K., Davison W. & Webster S.G.P. [1984]: *Ageing, the Facts,* Oxford University Press, Oxford).

chromosomes and genes. These may be due to template faults in DNA and RNA, possibly arising through mutations. Chemical mutagenic stimuli include hydroxy- and superoxide free radicals: physical stimuli include radiation.

5 The Hayflick limit

Cultured human embryonic fibroblasts appear to be capable of a maximum of 50 cell divisions give or take 10 either way. Towards the limit of their potential span, they acquire certain attributes of malignant cells, such as aneuploidy (varying chromosome numbers). Adult fibroblasts can only divide proportionally fewer times, and cells frozen for over 20 years 'remember' how many divisions they have left. The cellular redoubling capacity is never in fact reached because the organism ages and dies beforehand. Some individuals appear to enjoy enhanced cellular resistance with slower cell turnover so the Hayflick limit is reached later and there is a diminished risk of premature death. The biological clock of these 'biologically élite' individuals ticks by more slowly, and genetic factors do seem to play a significant part.

6 Immunological failure

Features of the immune system associated with ageing are:

(i) Cell-mediated immunity wanes, leading to a resurgence of tuberculosis and varicella (in the form of herpes zoster). Anergy (negative skin tests for example to tuberculin) is common.

(ii) Mucosal immunity probably declines.

(iii) There is a decline in humoral immunity (antibody production), but only to antigens requiring T helper cells due to thymic involution. This impairment of immune surveillance may impede the elimination of abnormal and neoplastic cells (Burnet).

(iv) Immunization to influenza remains effective but that to hepatitis seems to be less so.

(v) The T suppressor cells function less well, so auto-antibody production increases.

(vi) Malnutrition and diabetes are likely to compound these problems.

(vii) The neutrophil response seems less vigorous.

7 Colloid ageing

Chemical cross linkages develop between adjacent macromolecules, altering their physical properties. The changes have been compared with those easily detected between veal and beef, or in perished rubber and old glue or plastic. Some of these bridges are formed by disulphide bonds between suphydryl (SH) groups from cysteine, but recently attention has been directed to the non-enzymatic glycosylation of adjacent protein molecules. The resulting stiffening and loss of elasticity is reminiscent of the glycosylation of haemoglobin in diabetes and the ageing effects of that disease on the lens of the eye and the arteries.

8 Accumulation of waste products (the 'clinker' theory)

Intracellular lipofuscin granules can be found in nervous tissue, muscle, liver and kidney, especially in the elderly. Amyloid is a form of extracellular debris which also accumulates over the years, even in the absence of disease, and may affect organ function.

9 Defective homeostasis

A unifying hypothesis of the diminishing organ reserve and

increasing susceptibility to death which accompany ageing would be that the ageing physiology is characterized by an impaired ability to maintain a constant physical and chemical internal environment. Examples (see Chapter 15) include impaired glucose and drug metabolism, vulnerability to dehydration and hypothermia, and autonomic failure (Chapter 11). A minor insult is then sufficient to cause total breakdown, which may represent a mercifully brief final illness. A striking illustration of the lowered resistance that ensues was provided when it was recently shown that the area of burn required to yield a 50 per cent mortality rate (the LD 50) fell from 51 per cent in individuals aged 0–14 in the sample studied to only 9 per cent in those of 65 or over.

10 Genetic factors
Ageing must be at least partly genetically determined because animal species age at such different rates and the same changes occur 30 times faster in the mouse or rat than in man. Simple inherited abnormalities in man have drastic effects on ageing.

(a) Down's syndrome
A wide range of age-related pathologies appears prematurely.

(b) Werner's syndrome
This is due to a single autosomal recessive mutation. The following features of normal ageing are advanced by about 30 years:
  Whitening of hair
  Bilateral cataract
  Loss of subcutaneous tissue and muscle
  Progressive skin changes
  Atherosclerosis (the commonest cause of death, at about 46)
  Diabetes and cancers common
  Cells age more quickly *in vitro*

(c) Cockayne's syndrome
This is also an autosomal recessive condition with mental retardation and deafness, ataxia, retinal degeneration and optic atrophy. Premature ageing is displayed by cataracts, grey hair, atherosclerosis, limited joint movement and osteoporosis which may appear during the second year.

(d) Progeria
Although no clear genetic mechanism, it is mentioned here for

completeness. In addition to clinical features of ageing, there is a reduction in the number of cell doublings so that fibroblasts from a 19-year-old with this disease will reduplicate as many times as those from a normal person aged 60.

The fact that single genetic defects may have multiple effects on the individual's ageing may argue against multiple mechanisms of ageing and in favour of one basic cause.

Variability of ageing

The rate of ageing varies enormously between species if longevity is a valid index of ageing. Mice can live for 38 or possibly 40 months. The Carolina box-tortoise has been recorded as living for 129 years. The longest living mammal appears to be man, and no bird has been proved to live longer than 68, despite unconfirmed reports of much older cockatoos and vultures. Some fish may be capable of living well over a century but reliable data are lacking. The current authenticated record for a human is 117 (Japan) and this, like all records, is broken from time to time but not with regularity. It is interesting that this is so in view of the increasing number of individuals realizing their lifespan potential. In 1952, the Queen sent congratulatory messages to 200 UK citizens on reaching their 100th birthdays; in 1982 she despatched no fewer than 1750 similar missives.

The only experimentally substantiated prolongation of maximum life span has been achieved through dietary calorie restriction during the growth period. This has been repeatedly shown to be possible, using mainly rats and mice, over the past half century. Control mice have never lived longer than 44 months, but restricting calorie intake to 50 or 75 per cent of the ad lib consumption has extended life to over 54 months provided that dietary deficiencies are avoided. The shape of the survival curve is altered, and restricted animals are biologically younger than the controls, with postponement of diseases of ageing. It remains conceivable that such dietary restriction reproduces the more natural conditions experienced by rodents in the wild and that their life spans are being restored to those potentially possible under natural circumstances. However, the people of Okinawa seem to represent a human analogy, since they consume a complete although low calorie diet and enjoy a low incidence and late onset of the diseases of ageing

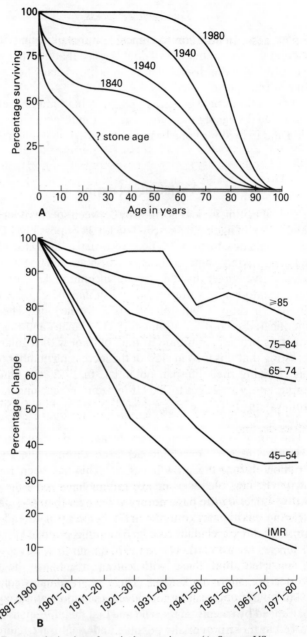

Fig. 4.2. Rectangularization of survival curves in man (**A:** Source: US Bureau of Health Statistics) and change in age-specific death rates in selected age groups in England and Wales (**B:** Source: Grundy E. [1984] Mortality and morbidity among the old. *British Medical Journal*, **288**, 663–4.)

and a far greater incidence of centenarians than does the rest of Japan.

Implications

In Chapter 2 attention was drawn to the growth in numbers of very old people anticipated in all countries during the next 2 or 3 decades. The human life span is not increasing but appears to be fixed at 110 to 120 years at most and the life expectancy is unlikely to exceed a maximum of 85 or so within the foreseeable future.

Commentators have described two radically different scenarios which might emerge from the trends described:

1 The optimistic view

The rectangularization of the survival curve. According to this view, the survival curve is becoming rectangular (see Fig. 4.2) as killing diseases are avoided or postponed and yet the life span remains fixed. The corollary is that older people will be much fitter. Health-conscious habits will ensure that the incidence of stroke and other disabling conditions continues to fall so that almost everyone can live until they reach the end of their natural lives, when homeostatic failure will bring about a mercifully swift final illness. The need for further massive investment in long-term care facilities will therefore decline.

2 The pessimistic view

Life expectancies of the older age groups have not increased as dramatically during the past century as have those at birth, but the increases in this country continue to be significant nevertheless. At the age of 85, life expectancy rose by 6 months (to 4.6 years for men and 5.6 years for women) between 1970–2 and 1978–80, and it has been suggested that those with chronic disabilities, including dementia, are surviving longer. The compression of morbidity expected by the optimists is not occurring, and there are cancers, arthritides and dementias whose aetiology and hence prevention remain elusive. Improved life expectancy in old age has not been accompanied by improved health expectancy. It may indeed be that the increasing life expectancy of old people consists of more years of disability and dependency than years of vigour and activity.

Conclusion

Research into human ageing should be accorded high priority because our present data base is totally inadequate for the formulation of health and fiscal policies. The research needs to be of high quality, and has in the past been bedevilled by the difficulty of distinguishing those observed decrements which are due to:

The ageing process itself

An increasing incidence of age-related diseases

Disuse phenomena associated with a less physically and mentally strenuous life-style

Further reading

Brody J.A. (1985) Prospects for an ageing population. *Nature,* **315,** 463–6.

Fries J.F. & Crapo L.M. (1981) *Vitality and Aging.* W.H. Freeman & Co., San Francisco.

Grundy E. (1984) Mortality and morbidity among the old (Leading article). *British Medical Journal,* **288,** 663–4.

Hayflick L. (1985) The cell biology of aging. *Clinics in Geriatric Medicine,* **I,** 15–27.

Holliday R. (1984) The aging process is a key problem in biomedical research. *Lancet,* **ii,** 1386–7.

Chapter 5
What's so Special about the Old?

Types of disease

The following categories of disease are frequently encountered:

1 Infections
Bacterial infections particularly involve the respiratory and urinary tracts. Cholecystitis, cellulitis, infective exacerbations of diverticular disease, septicaemia and infective arthritis and endocarditis are also common.

2 Degenerative disease
Atherosclerosis of the cerebral, coronary and peripheral arteries dominates the medicine of old age. Osteoarthritis is a major cause of pain and disability in the old. Alzheimer's disease (Chapter 7) poses the major challenge to the health and social services of the developed nations. Osteoporosis is causing a veritable epidemic of femoral neck fracture (Chapter 9).

3 Malignant disease
The common cancers are predominantly disorders of late life (Chapter 18).

4 Diminished organ reserve
Disease and environmental challenges readily disturb the precarious physiological equilibrium of the old (Chapter 15).

5 Chronic disability
Acute diseases require prolonged rehabilitation. Less acute ones tend to turn into long-term handicaps, especially if there are previous disabilities.

6 Deprivation-related health problems
Adverse social conditions have a major impact on health and well-being in old age.

Multiple pathology

It becomes inappropriate to attempt to explain all the symptoms, signs and abnormal investigation results in terms of a single disease process.

Altered presentation

Incontinence, confusion, falling and immobility have been described as the geriatric giants when describing the presentation of disease. Presentation is often non-specific, with pain sometimes poorly localized or absent and fever often less dramatic than in the young. Some pathologies are silent, others are quiet, and some doctors are not listening!

'Going off' or 'failure to thrive'

This syndrome may occur acutely, over a matter of hours or a day or two, when it is characterized by lethargy, confusion, taking to bed, incontinence, and failure to eat or drink (see Table 5.1). It may take a subacute course over a period of weeks or a month or two when the features will comprise diminished activity, mobility and self-care, falls, anorexia, weight loss, and perhaps confusion and aches and pains (see Table 5.2).

Table 5.1. Causes of 'going off'—hours/days

Abdominal crisis
Adverse drug reactions
Atrial fibrillation and other arrhythmia
Cardiac failure
Dehydration, electrolyte loss
Hypotension
Myocardial infarction
Pneumonia
Poisoning
Pulmonary thromboembolism
Respiratory failure
Septicaemia
Subdural haematoma
Urinary tract infection
Virus infections

Table 5.2. Causes of 'going off'—weeks/months

Addison's disease	Hypothyroidism
Alcohol	Infective endocarditis
Anaemia	Malabsorption
Atrial fibrillation	Malignancy
Carbon monoxide inhalation	Myopathy
Constipation	Parkinson's disease
Dementia	Polycythaemia
Depression	Polymyalgia rheumatica
Diabetes	Pyelonephritis
Drugs	Sleep apnoea
Gall bladder and biliary disease and other abdominal sepsis	Subdural haematoma
	Thyrotoxicosis
Gastric ulcer	Tuberculosis
Hypokalaemia	Uraemia
Hyponatraemia	Vitamin deficiency (including osteomalacia)

Non-self-referral

Many patients are brought to the attention of their doctors by relatives, neighbours or home-helps, and themselves have few complaints to offer. When kindly concern turns to deafening decibels, this becomes the familiar 'SMBD (Something Must Be Done—almost always by someone else) syndrome'.

The need to act fast

When old people are acutely ill, the physician must heed the advice given to Macbeth to 'be bloody, bold and resolute' if any contemplated intervention is to result in a patient restored to health and independence. When the illness is less life-threatening, it can still result in the long-term complications of immobility if effective treatment is not delivered promptly.

The problem-orientated approach

A list of problems as well as specific disease entities must be drawn up and addressed in order of priority.

The examination of the aged patient

Some departure from the classical medical model is mandatory if problems are to be adequately identified. Nebulous terms such as 'agility', 'frailty' and 'adverse power to weight ratio' are meaningful and justified. In the ward, a full assessment will probably be a two-or-three-stage procedure, especially if the patient is admitted acutely sick. It will not be appropriate to enquire details of the social background or administer a mental test score, or attempt to elicit the tendon reflexes before instituting resuscitative measures; all that can wait until the situation is much more stable.

Initial observation

1 Gait
Observe the gait as the patient enters; is it aided or unaided? Is it shuffling or unstable or a good firm stride? Note specific festinating, *petit pas*, stammering or foot-drop types of gait. Look for a shortened leg. Is there particular difficulty getting up and down from the chair?

2 Face
Look for a Parkinsonian demeanour (tremor may be absent), and for tardive dyskinesia which is so common especially in those on current or previous phenothiazine medication. Be receptive to the features of hypothyroidism or corticosteroid medication. Ptosis is common and its significance often doubtful. Look for signs of a facial weakness. Angular stomatitis is more often due to ill-fitting dentures than iron or vitamin deficiency. Vitiligo may be a pointer to auto-immune disorders.

3 Communication
Note any hearing difficulty—and be certain it is not a problem of comprehension. Note any visual disability.

4 The intellect
Is the conversation meaningful and appropriate? If so, the patient is probably orientated and has a reasonable grasp of her circum-stances. Questions should be relevant, for instance, who does the shopping is more important to the patient than the identity of the current prime minister. A mental test score should be administered to inpatients, when appropriate. An idea of the patient's premorbid mental and physical activity is important. A key question here is 'Do you fetch your pension?'

5 Physical examination

(i) Nutrition
Look for obesity, global wasting and signs of scurvy.

(ii) Neglect
Is the patient unkempt? Note particularly the state of the toenails and observe staining of clothing.

(iii) Kyphoscoliosis
This is a common finding and should be recorded.

(iv) Hydration
A little oedema does not necessarily mean that the patient is not basically dry, although absence of oedema may well do so. Conversely, it does not mean the patient is in heart failure. Beware the 'top and bottom' syndrome (puffy ankles, loss of tissue turgor in the upper trunk) and the 'in and out' syndrome (wet lungs, dry skin). These paradoxical situations arise due to difficulties in distribution of interstitial fluid, often denote an adverse prognosis, and lead to uncertainty as to whether the patient requires iv fluids or diuretics. Passing mention may be made of the 'geriatric paradoxes':
(a) A little oedema may be better than none.
(b) Check the blood pressure to ensure it is high enough.
(c) In some patients a little glycosuria is better than none.

The cardiovascular system
Extrasystoles are often numerous and hardly ever require treatment. The apex beat is commonly displaced but this may simply be due to kyphoscoliosis. Documentation of the peripheral pulses is very important in view of the prevalence of occult peripheral vascular disease (Chapter 12); in the absence of oedema, impalpable pulses are pathological. Bruits over carotid or femoral pulses are significant since an asymptomatic carotid bruit approximately doubles the risk of a stroke although even more patients will die from myocardial infarction. The blood pressure (Chapter 12) should ideally be measured both lying and standing.

The central nervous system

Note any tremor and whether accentuated by intention, rest or gravity. Note defective upward gaze—a very common finding and usually of uncertain significance. Absence of the corneal reflex has also been noted to be a fairly frequent finding. Apparent wasting of the hands can be misleading and of no significance. Contrary to popular belief, it is claimed that the ankle jerks, if patiently and methodically sought, should be present. They are often better elicited with the leg *straight*. Examine for tone, especially in the legs of those with walking difficulties. Note that hip disease must be excluded first.

The respiratory system

Be alert for Cheyne–Stokes respiration.

The abdomen

Beware the loaded colon. Consciously palpate and percuss for the bladder. Do a rectal examination to look for faecal impaction, tumour, prostate and pouch of Douglas.

Locomotor

Deliberately seek evidence of hip disease—there is a lot of it about. Likewise, painful restriction of shoulder and neck movement is common and disabling. Good grip strength and muscle bulk are non-specific favourable features.

Some ethical dilemmas in the medicine of old age

These are important but do not offer a right or wrong solution. Some of the authors' personal views are summarized:

1 Euthanasia

In the sense of enabling death to occur with minimal suffering and loss of dignity in the face of irreversible disease, we are in favour. We remain totally opposed to the deliberate termination of life.

2 How aggressively to investigate and treat the aged

The decision depends on the individual patient, but if there is any doubt, she should be given the benefit of it. No one should be denied access to technology on grounds of age alone.

3 Can research on the physically and mentally frail be justified?
Only if it is scientifically sound and ethical. It is morally unjustified
to withhold research which may benefit the elderly.

4 The NHS
The old are competing for resources with younger people with
family commitments. The old have contributed to the welfare state
through taxes and work.

5 Confidentiality of information
Sharing information with the team of health care practitioners is of
enormous benefit to the patient, for example at case conferences.

6 If one suspects abuse, should the might of the law be invoked?
Seldom—there are much better ways of relieving the situation
(Chapter 3).

7 The patient's interests conflict with those of the family
The reader's decision to purchase this book indicates that he/she
possesses, or soon will, the wisdom of Solomon!

Chapter 6
Disability and Rehabilitation

Definition

Rehabilitation comprises:
- Restoration to full activity after a severe illness (e.g. abdominal surgery, myocardial infarction).
- Restoration of maximum function following a specific impairment (e.g. stroke, fractured femoral neck).
- Facilitating the achievement of as much independence as possible despite continuing disability (e.g. Parkinson's disease, amputation, partially recovered stroke, hip disease).

Who does it?

Table 6.1. The rehabilitation team

Patient	Rehabilitation professions (physiotherapists, occupational therapists, speech therapists, appliance officers)	Chiropodist
Family	Voluntary workers	Social worker
Nurses and health visitors	Clinical psychologist	Doctor

Rehabilitation from acute illness

Hospital admission is often required, not for specific investigations or medication that cannot be administered at home, but because the weakness associated with a chest infection or heart disease renders the patient unable to attend to her bodily needs and fluid intake. She may feel too unwell to get out of bed for a day or two. Unless there is adequate support at home, admission needs to be arranged without delay, otherwise pressure sores, contractures, constipation, incontinence and loss of confidence are inevitable and will necessitate protracted rehabilitation. Remobilization is achieved by suitable exercises (passive, assisted, resisted) combined with functional exercise such as transfers, sitting to standing, and walking. Activities of daily living (ADL) abilities are assessed and various items of equipment may be deployed to facilitate independence. Following discharge, the able-bodied may consider positive measures to promote physical fitness.

Stroke

See also Chapter 10; the following stages can be recognized in the recovery from a stroke:

1 The initial phase
In those who are seriously ill, treatment is directed at the care of the unconscious or clouded patient. Attention is given to the airway, the pressure areas, hydration (iv or rectally), the bladder and the prevention of infection.

2 Return to the world
The patient is propped up to restore contact with the world and to protect the lungs. Early attention from the speech therapist is required for the dysphasic, dysarthric and also for the dysphagic patient. A fine-bore nasogastric tube may be necessary in the short term, and so may a urinary catheter. The persistently hemianopic patient who cannot compensate for this disability is placed so that the intact field of vision embraces real life and not a blank wall. Patients with hemianopia need to be made aware of the lost field of vision and to be taught to search it out by turning the eyes and the head. If this is not done early on, they are likely to remain unaware of obstacles to the affected side. The physiotherapist proceeds with the sequence of remobilization previously outlined. The medical staff can define the precise extent of the neurological deficit, and should assess the degree of cognitive impairment, if any, as well as seeking evidence of inattention, loss of body image, disordered spatial perception and other parietal signs.

3 Participation in the world
The sequence of sitting, transferring, standing and walking mark the fundamental steps in recovery, and in patients with an initially severe hemiplegia usually take a couple of months or thereabouts.

The physiotherapist pays almost as much attention to the un-
affected side and adopts a bilateral approach. The ideal is to avoid
as far as possible unilateral aids such as tripods which may per-
petuate poor balance. Symmetrical movements are more natural
and help to reduce spasticity. The occupational therapist con-
centrates on vital ADL such as dressing and using the toilet. Should
this stage take place in a stroke unit? Current evidence suggests
that these units contribute to our knowledge of stroke disease, may
yield short-term functional results, but probably produce little
long-term benefit over and above the geriatric or general medical
wards. Does any of this activity need to take place as an inpatient at
all? The main reason for admission of the stroke patient is that he or
she is initially too ill and too dependent to be looked after at home,
taking into account the support available.

4 Back to the real world

Grooming for discharge includes finding out how much the patient
will need to do, how much she can do, and what 'prostheses' (e.g.
home-helps and appliances) can be supplied to perform for her
those tasks she and her spouse (if any) cannot do. Adaptations to
the home may be required. Following discharge, further improve-
ments may continue for at least a year and may be assisted by
continued formal rehabilitation for a time in a day hospital or by
membership of a stroke club (see Chapter 10 and Table 6.2).

Table 6.2. Outcome of stroke survivors (community surveys)

	Percentage
Full or almost full function	25–50
Able to return to work (of those working before)	29–36
Unable to walk outdoors	41
Unable to walk without assistance	20–27
Of those who walk, require an aid	66
Dependent in some aspect of self-care	31–52
Long-term institution	12–21

(Source: Langton–Hewer R. (1984) Recovery from stroke. In:
Grimley Evans J. & Caird F.I. (eds) *Advanced Geriatric Medicine 4.*
London, Pitman Publishing, pp. 201–9)

Barriers to successful rehabilitation:

- Global impairment of higher cerebral function.
- Poor motivation (patient or carers).

- Depression.
- Communication difficulties.
- Sensory deprivation.
- Associated pathology (arthritis, heart failure).
- Pressure sores, contractures.
- Loss of body image, sensory ataxia.
- Persistent swallowing difficulty.
- Unrealistic expectations.

General rules regarding stroke

1 Early adverse prognostic features for survival include loss of consciousness, respiratory abnormalities, conjugate deviation of the eyes, and atrial fibrillation. A poor functional outcome can be predicted in the presence of incontinence, hemianopia, poor sitting balance with severe motor deficit, parietal signs, and especially intellectual impairment.

2 Life expectancy is greatly reduced.

3 Recurrence is common but most die of heart disease.

4 Dysphasia—most recover but recovery is less likely if dysphasia is severe at 6 months, although in a few cases more rapid progress is made during the second 6 months.

5 Incontinence—if lasting for 8 weeks with a serious intellectual deficit, it will be permanent. Fifty per cent recover in 6 months.

6 Proximal movements recover first and legs fare better than arms.

7 Muscle power has returned about as far as it is likely to at 3 months, but perhaps a further 10 per cent recovery continues to take place between 3 and 12 months.

8 Useful function of the arm is unlikely if improvement has not occurred after 1 month.

Effectiveness of therapy

The current 'gold standard' is the Northwick Park trial published in 1981 in which 133 outpatients were randomized into three groups:

(i)   Intensive—4 whole days per week.

(ii) Conventional—3 half days per week.

(iii) No formal therapy, but general support and encouragement. When measured by ADL score, those in group 1 improved faster and more than those in group 2, who in turn did better than those in group 3. More patients in group 3 subsequently relapsed than in the other 2 groups.

Fracture of the femoral neck

The aim of the surgeon with regard to the fracture is to 'fix it and forget it'. If it has been securely fixed, the patient can weight bear as soon as her general condition permits, which usually means starting the day after the operation. In an ideal world, pre- and post-operative medical attention would be shared with the geriatric department in those patients who are rather more complex, being generally older and afflicted by more pathology. Rehabilitation would be undertaken in a geriatric-orthopaedic ward, since, although figures confirming improved results are difficult to obtain, there seems to be little doubt that collaboration between the two departments is beneficial. The outcome is influenced by a number of factors, particularly prompt surgery and premorbid physical, nutritional and mental status.

The amputee

There are two major factors likely to influence the outcome favourably:
1 The patient should be in good general condition and the remaining limb must not have a heel sore, even though the odds are high that it is ischaemic. Hence—amputation should be offered as a positive procedure rather than as a last resort after many weeks of morphine-clouded misery.
2 The stump must heal satisfactorily. Hence it is important to amputate at a high enough level. It remains true, nationwide, that the majority of operations are above-knee (AK) which is much quicker, although some centres manage to perform two-thirds of their amputations below-knee (BK). About 40–50 per cent of AK amputees walk, compared with 80 per cent of BK amputees.

Procedure

1 Within a few days, commence bandaging to shape the stump correctly. At the same time passive and then active stump exercises are started.
2 Walking between parallel bars and then with sticks, tetrapod or frame restores balance.
3 As soon as oedema has settled and healing is satisfactory (usually at about 7 days), the patient is measured for a prosthesis. An

inflatable prosthesis can be used at 5 or 7 days. A pylon is a very useful temporary appliance and can often be fitted 2 weeks postoperatively.

4 The patient becomes not only ambulant with the definitive prosthetic limb, but also adept at putting it on, locking it, taking it off.

5 Grooming for discharge includes nursing instruction in stump care, assessment and practice in ADL activities and adaptation of the home.

Reasons for failure to rehabilitate after amputation

1 Dementia, depression, refusal.
2 Stump presents insuperable technical problems.
3 Cardiovascular or muscular insufficiency.
4 Severe ischaemia or pressure affecting other limb.
5 Other pathology—stroke, arthritis.

If it is clear that it is unrealistic to expect the patient to become ambulant again, a positive decision must be taken to aim for wheelchair independence.

Parkinson's disease

How can you 'rehabilitate' from an irreversible and progressive disease? Physical treatment has three main places in the management of the disorder:

1 In the early case as the first line of treatment.
2 Rehabilitation after a fall, a fracture, or a period of immobility necessitated by severe systemic illness, all of which will cause a profound decline in functional state.
3 In combination with levodopa therapy as an ongoing attempt to delay the progress of the disease. If the condition is stable, there is doubt concerning the value of maintenance physical therapy: perhaps 'pulses' of treatment are more useful.

Disability

Depending on one's definition, 60–75 per cent of disabled people in the community are over 65. Among persons over 80, probably about 30 per cent have become housebound, often due to specific disabilities but quite often having abruptly withdrawn from the outside world after some event which has subtly cloaked their self-perception with the mantle of infirmity. Such events include a hospital admission, a bereavement, a fall in a public place. Some results of a recent local community survey are given in Table 6.3.

Table 6.3. Disabilities among 1121 East Anglians aged 75 and over

Function	%
Unable to cook main meals	35
Unable to shop	35
Difficulty getting about home	24
Difficulty with stairs or steps	50
Unable to do stairs/steps at all or only with help	19
Need help cutting toenails	44
Medium or high dependency due to visual loss	8
Medium or high dependency through hearing loss	7.5
Incontinence of urine	13

(Source: Kemp F. (1985) Survey of the Elderly at Home, *Occasional Paper 14*. Department of Community Medicine, University of Cambridge)

Further reading

Caird F.I., Kennedy R.D. & Williams B.O. (1983) *Practical Rehabilitation of the Elderly*. Pitman, London.

Chapter 7
The Ageing Brain

Age changes

1 Neuronal loss
The daily neuronal loss through life is estimated at $50-100 \times 10^3$ out of an original total of 10^{9-11}. This fallout affects cerebral and cerebellar cortex and locus caeruleus but not the nuclei of the pons or medulla. It also occurs in lower mammals. It is crudely reflected in a decrease in brain weight.

2 Lipofuscin accumulation
Present in both neurons and glial cells (see Chapter 4).

3 Loss of synapses
This has been demonstrated in the cortex of ageing rats and affects the pyramidal cells.

4 Glial cell proliferation
This does not occur uniformly but seems to affect the hippocampus more than the neocortex.

5 Neurotransmitter function
The cholinergic system has been extensively investigated, and there seems to be a slight decline in choline acetyl transferase (CAT) activity in the cortex and the caudate nucleus. Catecholamine, serotonin and GABA function have been less fully studied and results have been less consistent.

6 Cerebral blood flow and metabolic rate
Those studies which purport to show a decline have been criticized for failure to select representative subjects.

Psychology of ageing

Memory and cognitive function

Intelligence testing, learning ability, short-term memory and reaction time decline with age as tested by cross-sectional studies. There is usually a greater scatter than with younger subjects, partly due to a greater prevalence of sensory, motor or cognitive impairment.

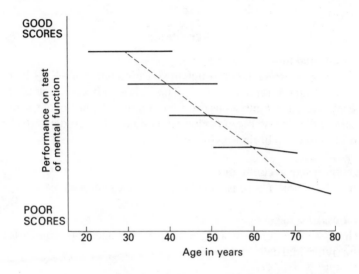

Fig. 7.1. Different age cohorts are reassessed 7 and 14 years after initial testing: younger cohorts begin at a higher level ('succeeding generations are brighter'), so cross-sectional comparisons (dashed line) give an exaggerated impression of mental deterioration with advancing age. (Source: Huppert F.A. [1982] Does mental function decline with age. *Geriatric Medicine* **XII**, 32–37).

Different generations have different educational and life experiences so longitudinal studies (Fig. 7.1) tend to show the decline often does not become significant until the age of 75 or so. With regard to memory it is usually retrieval that becomes impaired more than assimilation or storage, perhaps because of the mass of data to be sorted. Although not universal, 'benign senescent forgetfulness' is certainly very common.

Emotion and personality
The stereotyped image is of increasing introversion, disengagement and pessimism, but there is little firm evidence to suggest that these are inevitable accompaniments of ageing, despite societal expectations.

Sleep
Sleep appears to deteriorate in many ways as we grow old and the more important are shown below:

Complaints of insomnia ↑ (26–45 per cent)
Time in bed ↑
Time actually spent sleeping ↓
Number and duration of awakenings ↑
Stage 4 sleep period ↓
Rapid eye movement (REM) sleep ↓

Complaints of insomnia are frequent and possible causes should be sought. They include the following:

Anxiety
Depression
Pain
Discomfort due to constipation
Urgency, frequency, nocturia
Restless legs (Chapter 11)
Cramps
Daytime napping
Nocturnal cough
Unrealistic expectations

If no cause is apparent the problem may be solved by simple advice:

Rising at a regular and early hour
Maintain activity during the day
Avoid coffee or tea during the evening
Do not go to bed hungry
Warm milky drink
Cold alcoholic drink
Do not go to bed too early

If hypnotics are resorted to, a course of 3 or 4 weeks is recommended as prolonged administration may lead to somnolence, confusion, unsteadiness and habituation. Specific sleep disorders include snoring and sleep apnoea (Chapter 13).

The failing brain

Acute brain failure: confusional states, delirium

Organic illness can cause acute confusion at any age but the old are particularly vulnerable and those with underlying chronic brain failure especially so. The clinical features are given below:

Onset typically abrupt

Marked variability: lucid intervals

Consciousness clouded

Impaired recent memory

Disorientation in place and time

Delusions and hallucinations

Fear, bewilderment, restlessness

Possibly—signs of underlying cause

The following causes should be considered:

Intracranial

Infarction —'silent'—often frontal

Infection —Meningo-encephalitis

Injury —head injury, fat embolism

Iatrogenic —drugs acting on CNS

Extracranial

Infection —especially pulmonary and urinary

Metabolic —fluid and electrolyte imbalance, hypoglycaemia, hypothermia

Anoxia —cardiac or respiratory failure

Toxic —alcohol, drugs

Nutritional —Wernicke's encephalopathy

Treatment is summarized as follows:

1 Plentiful reassurance and explanation and avoidance of argument.

2 Treat underlying cause.

3 Attend to fluid and electrolyte balance.

4 Attention to nutrition—give Parentrovite if in doubt.

5 Nocturnal restlessness—use chlormethiazole or thioridazine.

6 Daytime restlessness—use thioridazine or haloperidol up to 30 mg per day.

Chronic brain failure: dementia

Definition

Dementia is a global impairment of the intellect, memory and personality without any alteration of conscious level.

Prevalence

Approximately 2 per cent of people between 65 and 75, rising to 20 per cent over the age of 80, suffer from significant dementia (Fig. 7.2). These figures seem to be the best information we have at present, although some evidence is emerging that they may be overestimates.

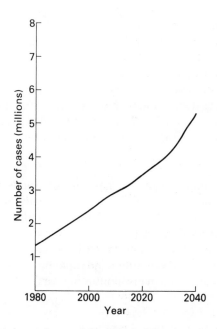

Fig. 7.2. Predicted prevalence of dementia in USA assuming stable age-specific prevalence (Source: Cross P. & Garland G.J. [1986] *The Epidemiology of Dementing Disorders,* Office of Technology Assessment, Washington).

Types of dementia

The dementias can be divided into senile dementia of Alzheimer type (SDAT or simply AD) (55 per cent), multi-infarct dementia (15 per cent), mixed dementia (20–25 per cent), and comparatively rarely, dementia secondary to the other organic diseases given below:

Drugs—alcohol, barbiturates

Trauma—subdural haematoma (Chapter 11)

B_{12} deficiency—'megaloblastic madness'

Hypothyroidism—'myxoedema madness'
Syphilis
Normal pressure hydrocephalus (triad of dementia, ataxia, incontinence)
Malignant disease—non-metastatic
Intracranial space occupying lesion (SOL)

Diagnosis of dementia
The diagnosis of a dementing process is often difficult, and the following points should be borne in mind:
1 The necessity to be certain that a bizarre lifestyle is not simply due to eccentricity. Self-neglect, in particular, is not always due to intellectual impairment.
2 The patient may volunteer a history of failing memory. This sometimes causes depression—or may be the result of depression.
3 A mental test score (Fig. 7.3) should be administered, but not necessarily as soon as the patient is admitted. Caution is needed in interpreting the result, especially in the deaf, depressed, drugged or dying.
4 A physical examination may suggest a possible underlying cause.
5 In the absence of physical signs or headache, computed tomography (CT) of the head is probably only indicated in:
(a) those under 65–70 years of age
(b) those in their late sixties or early seventies in whom the dementia is clearly of recent onset and rapid progression (weeks or a few months rather than many months or years).

Clinical features
The clinical features of SDAT are outlined below:
> Depression common in early stages
> Capacity for abstract thought progressively impaired
> Reduced learning ability, loss of initiative
> Loss of concentration and interest, aimlessness
> Poor memory (initially short-term then long-term)
> Behaviour disinhibited, noisy, antisocial or aggressive
> Deteriorating standards of hygiene
> Restlessness, wandering
> Confusion, disorientation
> Parietal and other neurological signs
> Incontinence

MENTAL TEST SCORE

PATIENT'S NAME ....

AGE: ....

DATE: ....

1. Name?							
2. Occupation?							
3. Married?							
4. Address?							
5. Date .... Year .... Month ..... Day							
6. Where are you now? (Tell patient if he/she does not know and ask again at the end of the test.)							
7. Ask patient to remember this address 79 Columbia Rd (Ask patient to repeat it to you then, and again at the end of test.)							
8. Prime Minister?							
9. Name of Queen?							
10. Where is Belfast?							
11. What is happening there at the moment?							
12. Date of 2nd World War (years)							
13. Prime Minister at beginning of it?							
8 – Poor 12 – Good							
SCORE:							
OTHER QUESTIONS e.g. Proverbs. Serial 7's Flowers Colours							
SCORE:							

One mark each question (NO ½ MARKS)

Fig. 7.3. Card for mental test score.

Apathy, inability to converse or engage attention, blunted emotion

Repetitive speech or movement

Dysphasia

Epilepsy (in 5–10 per cent)

Physical dependency

Pathology and aetiology

The following are the main pathological features of SDAT:

1 Thinning of cortex, dilated sulci and ventricles.
2 Grossly increased loss of cortical neurones in temporal lobes and hippocampus.
3 Gross increase in neuritic plaques in cortex containing a core of amyloid protein: cerebrovascular amyloid deposits are also found.
4 Gross increase in neurofibrillary tangles consisting of paired helical filaments possibly derived from aberrant protein.
5 CAT activity reduced throughout cortex and nucleus basalis.
6 Somatostatin and corticotropin releasing factor somewhat reduced—mainly temporal lobe: gamma amino butyric acid deficit.
7 Loss of cortical input by projection fibres due to cell loss in nucleus basalis (cholinergic) and locus caeruleus (noradrenergic).
Suggested aetiological factors include:
    Slow virus
    Auto-immune mechanism
    Aluminium accumulation
    Genetic basis (it is occasionally transmitted as a single gene autosomal dominant and appears prematurely in Down's syndrome). The gene conferring susceptibility and that transmitting familial AD are located on chromosome 21 in proximity to the gene carrying amyloid protein
    Association with Parkinson's disease (Chapter 11)
    The pathology and aetiology of multi-infarct disease are relatively straightforward. Multiple cerebral infarction is due to arterial disease and its familiar causes: dementia seems to result when cortical or subcortical softenings total a volume of 50–100 ml.

Management of dementia

Specific therapy for SDAT remains the elusive 'crock of gold', although at the time of writing, increasingly encouraging results are reported from cholinergic agents such as centrally active anticholinesterases. Until these observations are translated into clinical practice, there remain several vital functions which the doctor must fulfil:
1 He must establish the diagnosis and exclude treatable conditions and counsel the family accordingly.
2 He should support the supporters: domiciliary services, day care, holiday relief, the psychiatric community nurse, the Alzheimer's Disease Society are all important sources of relief.
3 Symptoms may need controlling—constipation, insomnia,

hallucinations, agitation and restlessness will often require appropriate measures (see acute brain syndrome).

4 Advice will eventually be necessary concerning temporary or permanent institutional care and what type is most suitable.

5 Whether at home or in an institution, the patient's orientation should be positively promoted ('reality orientation').

6 The doctor has a responsibility to ensure that certain legal requirements are complied with. They include the following:

(a) Testamentary capacity and power of attorney

The patient should know the nature of the action of making a will, have a reasonable grasp of the extent of her assets, know the persons to whom she may leave her property, and be free of delusions which might distort her judgement. Otherwise, she is 'incapable by reason of mental disorder of managing and administrating her property and affairs'. Until recently, loss of testamentary capacity automatically invalidated any power of attorney. It still precludes arranging one, but there is now an 'Enduring Power of Attorney' (1985) which is initiated while of sound mind but, if registered with the Court of Protection when the donor is mentally incapable, endures thereafter.

(b) Court of protection

Normally, any patient who has a moderate estate, but who is not of testamentary capacity, should have her affairs placed in the hands of the Court of Protection. Application may be made by a relative, the solicitor, or the doctor.

(c) Compulsory committal

This is only ever used as a last resort.

MENTAL HEALTH ACT, 1983

Section 2—Admission for assessment
• Applicant—nearest relative or approved social worker.
• Signatories—two doctors—one must know the patient (preferably GP) and the other having special experience.
• Duration—28 days.

Section 3—Admission for treatment. Up to 6 months, unless consultant discharges patient sooner.

Section 4—Emergency admission
- Applicant—as above—must have seen patient within 24 hours.
- Signatory—any doctor.
- Duration—72 hours.

Section 5—Holding power. Informal patients may be forcibly detained for up to 6 hours by a qualified mental illness nurse if the doctor is not available. The consultant or his deputy may enforce the detention for 72 hours.

Section 7—Guardianship. This is more widespread in Canada and the USA than in this country. On the grounds of mental disorder and in the interests of the patient's welfare, a guardian may be appointed who can cause her to reside in a given place, attend for treatment, and allow access to a doctor or approved social worker.
- Applicant—nearest relative or approved social worker.
- Signatories—2 registered practitioners.
- Guardian—Local Social Services Authority or any other person.
- Duration—14 days.

NATIONAL ASSISTANCE ACT

Section 47—Removal to place of safety. This section applies more to the physically infirm than the mentally disordered, particularly if in danger through self-neglect or if endangering others. The GP may apply to the community physician for compulsory removal to a geriatric or psycho-geriatric ward or to a local authority residential home. The authority of a magistrate is required and the duration is 3 weeks. The section is intended to enforce removal when it is likely that this will substantially improve the patient's health. It is often initiated by a social worker.

Self-neglect

Old people are not infrequently encountered living in conditions of extreme degradation with total disregard of hygiene and self-care. A sub-group of this 'senile squalor syndrome' are those who are not in any way demented and who hoard vast quantities of rubbish, and this has been termed the Diogenes syndrome. This condition may lead to hypothermia, malnutrition and infestation, and there are several risk factors:

Dementia
Depression
Bereavement and isolation
Poverty
Disability
Alcohol
Previous psychiatric disorder
Mental subnormality
Lifelong difficult personality/eccentricity

Alcoholism

The prevalence of old-age alcoholism is unknown but two groups are recognized. Group 1 are the 'graduate' heavy drinkers who survive into old age, despite the odds against. Numbers of men and women are similar. Complications include hallucinations, Wernicke's encephalopathy, dementia, falls, and self-neglect. Group 2 are the 'late onset' drinkers who take to the habit to assuage loneliness and ill-health. Women outnumber men 5 to 1, and depression is a common association in addition to the complications noted above. The decision to treat entails total withdrawal and should delirium tremens ensue, it is controlled with chlormethiazole.

Hallucinations

Hallucinations are common in the aged and remain of uncertain significance. Probable associations are given below but sometimes no cause can be found:

Eye pathology
Bereavement
Depression
Acute brain syndrome (including drugs)
Dementia
Other psychiatric disorders (alcohol, chronic schizophrenia)

Depression

Prevalence in persons over 65
Community surveys have shown rates of 10–15 per cent.

Special features
An underlying physical disease is very common. The illness is usually unipolar, and apathy, withdrawal and self-neglect frequently lead to a suspicion of dementia ('pseudo dementia'). There is a high suicide risk and the age-specific mortality rises steadily well into advanced old age, particularly in men over 80 (200 per million population): the elderly account for a third of all suicides. Unsuccessful suicide attempts, on the other hand, seem to be less common than in younger age groups. The usual clinical features of depression are often not very dissimilar to those in other age groups:

Apathy, withdrawal, loss of interest
Anxiety or agitation
Delusions of disease, guilt or poverty
Sleep disturbance
Loss of appetite, dehydration, constipation
Sadness, dread, hopelessness

Treatment

1 Supportive. Includes counselling and relief of loneliness.

2 Drugs. It is important to start with a low dose, and if the patient responds, treatment is maintained for 3 months and then tailed off gradually under supervision. The tricyclic compounds, in particular, cause numerous adverse reactions but dothiepin seems to be relatively non-toxic. The serotonin receptor inhibitor trazodone may prove to be preferable.

3 Electroconvulsive therapy (ECT). This has had a bad press but may be life saving in elderly depressives who fail to respond to antidepressants. It is usually well tolerated although confusion and memory impairment may ensue.

Schizophrenia

This, like problem-drinking can be divided into 'graduate' and 'late onset' schizophrenia (paraphrenia). Paranoid delusions are common and treatment is with a major tranquillizer (e.g. chlorpromazine).

Neurosis

Institutional
This condition is iatrogenic and should thus be preventable. It has been called 'the mental pressure sore'.

Anxiety
Anxiety is very common in older people, and may accompany depression, dementia and physical illness—or may cause physical symptoms (palpitations, breathlessness, giddiness, abdominal discomfort, bowel fixation). Treatment is by reassurance or minor tranquillizers, if necessary.

Further reading

Anon (1987) Alzheimer's disease, Down's syndrome and chromosome 21. *Lancet*, **i,** 1011–12.

Arie T. (ed.) (1985) *Recent Advances in Psychogeriatrics*, Vol. 1. Churchill Livingstone, Edinburgh.

Cybulska E. (1986) Gross self-neglect in old age. *British Journal of Hospital Medicine*, **36,** 21–5.

Mulley G.P. (1986) Differential diagnosis of dementia. *British Medical Journal*, **292,** 1416–8.

Roth M. & Iversen L.L. (eds) (1986) *British Medical Bulletin*, Vol. 42, no. 1. Churchill Livingstone, Edinburgh.

Chapter 8
Falls and Immobility

Falls

Falls in old age are common, important, dangerous and usually a symptom of a serious underlying problem.

Frequency of falls

In one year one-third of old people in their own homes will experience a fall. Women fall more frequently than men; the old old fall more frequently than the young old; the very old (over 85) fall less frequently, probably due to reduced activity or survival of the super fit; the institutionalized elderly fall most frequently of all.

Principal causes of recurrent falls

Isolated falls are very common in any systemic illness. Recurrent falls have a large variety of causes:

1 Age-related
(i) Body sway increases with age—impaired compensatory mechanisms lead to more frequent falls. Body sway in women is always greater than in men—at all ages.
(ii) Walking patterns become less efficient and more irregular— will be made worse by unsuitable footwear and neurological disease.

2 Environment-related
(i) The elderly tend to live in the oldest and worst accommodation.
(ii) Their living accommodation is sometimes cluttered, e.g. with walking frames, flexes, rugs and pets.
(iii) Unfamiliar environment increases risks, e.g. on admission to an institution or move to new accommodation.

3 Impaired sensory input
(i) Visual impairment (cataracts, glaucoma, inappropriate or dirty glasses) makes detection of hazards difficult.
(ii) Impaired hearing and balance, including vertigo and dizziness.
(iii) Peripheral neuropathy makes walking difficult and potentially dangerous.

4 Drug-related
(i) Sedatives impair insight and balance.
(ii) Postural hypotension often iatrogenic.
(iii) Cardiac dysrhythmias may be iatrogenic.

5 Locomotor disorders
(i) In neurological impairment, e.g. Parkinson's disease, residual effects of stroke, peripheral neuropathy.
(ii) With joint disorders, e.g. pain and deformity in osteoarthritis.
(iii) Muscle abnormality, e.g. proximal myopathy.

6 Fall in cerebral perfusion
(i) Cardiac—rate and rhythm changes and inability to maintain steady blood pressure.
(ii) Cerebrovascular—transient brain stem ischaemia.
(iii) Syncope—secondary to cough, micturition, carotid sinus, aortic stenosis.
(iv) Drop attacks—see Chapter 11.

7 Epilepsy

Investigation of falls

History—was it a trip or a 'funny turn'?
1 A trip = no impairment of consciousness
   The patient can usually explain away the episode (but beware—frequent and regular falls are rarely accidental)
   The patient is often 'young old' and is usually in reasonable health
   Underlying cause is likely to be found in Sections 2, 3, 4 or 5 of the above list
2 'Turn' = there may be a warning sensation
   Consciousness may be lost
   The patient is puzzled by the event
   The patient is likely to be 'old old', i.e. older than 75 years

The patient is likely to be generally frail

Causes are usually found in the above list in Sections 6 or possibly 4

NB   Obtain other information from other witnesses; take drug history.

Examination
Must be complete and thorough but pay particular attention to:
1 Pulse rate and rhythm; massage the carotid sinus.
2 Blood pressure—standing and lying.
3 Source of emboli—murmurs, bruits.
4 Central nervous system lateralizing signs.
5 Evidence of Parkinson's disease.
6 Myxoedema.
7 Peripheral neuropathy.
8 Proximal myopathy.
9 Vision and hearing.
10 Neck movements.
11 Mental test score.

Helpful tests
1 Haemoglobin? polycythaemia or anaemia—proceed to find cause.
2 Electrolytes and blood sugar, if abnormal, pursue cause.
3 ECG—Standard leads—? infarction ?conduction defect,
24-hour monitoring if dysrhythmia suspected.
4 Thyroid function tests—thyroid disease can be very occult in the elderly.
5 Seek underlying infection—chest X-ray, mid-stream urine and blood cultures.
6 Cerebral blood flow; scan if multi-infarct disease suspected.
7 If fits suspected—EEG, CT scan in selected cases.

Treatment
1 Identifiable causes or contributing factors—treat appropriately.
2 No cause found—reduce risks from falls:
(i) Maintain constant environmental temperature.
(ii) Soften floor coverings, i.e. carpet rooms.
(iii) Remove obstacles and dangers, e.g. guard fire.
(iv) Place emergency bedding in position where it can be reached from the floor.

(v) Arrange for alarm system or frequent visitors.
(vi) Teach how to get up from the floor without help.

Complications of falls

These may be divided into those related to the fall (see below) and those due to lying on the floor (see immobility).

1 Physical injury
(i) Soft tissue bruising—may require analgesics if mobility is to be maintained. May be reflected in raised muscle enzyme levels.
(ii) Break in skin may be very slow to heal and grafting may be required.
(iii) Fractures, orthopaedic treatment may be required.
(iv) Pressure sores 'can occur after a long lie' (see Chapter 19).
(v) Friction burn from synthetic carpet on attempting to get up.
(vi) Fall on to a fire or a hot surface, e.g. radiator may result in a burn.
(vii) Hypothermia may result if fall occurs in the cold, e.g. outside or in an unheated room (see Chapter 15).

2 Psychological injury
(i) Loss of confidence and mobility—may result in becoming housebound.
(ii) Anxiety/depression about the future.

3 Social injury
(i) Because of intolerable anxiety in carers (formal and informal).
(ii) Increased demands on carer may cause antagonism.
(iii) Need to move to safer surroundings may separate faller from current supporters.

4 Death
(i) As direct consequence of the fall.
(ii) Up to 25 per cent of frequent fallers are dead within one year of presentation, not directly due to injuries but because of underlying cause of falls.

Immobility

Over half of all elderly people over 75 years of age (53 per cent) have difficulty in getting around their own home. Twenty per cent are totally housebound and most find it difficult to climb on to a bus and are also unable to drive.

Reasons for immobility are

(i) Pain and stiffness in bones, joints and muscles (see Table 8.1).
(ii) Weakness, including generalized systemic disease (see Table 8.2).
(iii) Fear/anxiety/depression/dementia (see Table 8.3).
(iv) Frequent falls.
(v) Iatrogenic, e.g. sedation, surgery (amputations and unsuccessful orthopaedic procedures).

Table 8.1. Pain/stiffness as cause of immobility

In joints	In muscles	In bones
Osteoarthritis	Myositis	Osteoporosis
Rheumatoid arthritis	Polymyalgia rheumatica	Osteomalacia
Gout	Myxoedema	Paget's disease
Pseudogout	Parkinson's disease	Malignant disease
Infection		

Table 8.2. Weakness as cause of immobility

Neuronal damage	Muscle damage	Reduced effort tolerance
Hemiplegia	Disuse	Dyspnoea
Peripheral neuropathy	Myopathy	Anaemia
Motor neurone disease	Amyotrophy	Reduced cardiac output
Paraplegia	Hypokalaemia	

Table 8.3. Psychological causes of immobility

Fear and anxiety	—of falling
Manipulative behaviour	—to ensure attention
Depression	—apathy reduces initiative
Dementia	—reduces insight into need to maintain mobility and independence is neglected

(vi) Foot care disorders, e.g. bunions and nail abnormalities also severe ischaemia and infection.

Complications of immobility

1 Physical
Muscle wasting (see Chapter 9)
Osteoporosis (see Chapter 9)
Muscle contractures
Pressure sores (see Chapter 19)
Hypothermia (see Chapter 19)
Hypostatic pneumonia
Constipation
Incontinence
Deep vein thrombosis

2 Psychological
Depression
Loss of confidence

3 Social
Isolation

Fitness to drive

Every driver must realize that a time may come when they will have to surrender their driving licence. Ironically driving usually has to be abandoned when alternative methods of movement/travel become even more difficult. However, it should be remembered that the occasional use of taxis, etc. is more cost-effective than maintaining a rarely used car.

Vehicles may be modified to enable driving to continue in spite of disabilities and cars with automatic gears enable some disabled persons to continue to drive.

In the UK at the age of 70 years, a driver should consult his GP regarding ability to continue driving. The driving licence must be renewed at the age of 70 and at 3-year intervals on declaration of good health.

The following will render a patient unfit to drive:
1 Recurrent episodes of cerebral ischaemia.
2 Episodic changes in level of consciousness, e.g. due to blood

pressure changes or significant vertigo, or poorly controlled diabetes mellitus.

3 Paroxysms of cardiac arrhythmia and severe ischaemic heart disease.

4 Severe Parkinson's disease.

5 Fluctuating or progressively declining intellectual ability.

6 Uncorrectable visual impairment.

NB   Accident rates for drivers begin to increase after the age of 55 years.

Advice for elderly drivers

1 Concentrate—do not be diverted by conversation or radio.

2 Drive for short periods with regular rests, i.e. avoid fatigue.

3 Prepare your route well and allow plenty of time for the journey.

4 Avoid peak traffic times and night driving.

5 Pay particular attention when starting, stopping and changing direction.

Fitness to fly

1 The partial pressure of oxygen falls at high altitude, even in pressurized aircraft. The 3 per cent reduction in saturization of arterial blood can be significant to patients with severe cardio-respiratory disease, and patients with a haemoglobin level of less than 8.8 g. Supplementary oxygen during flight will compensate.

2 Dehydration may occur because of the reduced humidity at high altitudes—fluid intake must therefore be maintained.

3 Extra space may be required by passengers with disabilities; this may be particularly important on economy flights.

4 Patients with mobility problems may not be able to cope (unassisted) with the arrangement of space at airports.

5 Post-operative patients, up to 10 days after abdominal or chest surgery, may run into difficulties because of gas expansion (e.g. in gut or pleural space) at high altitudes.

6 Colostomies may function, more frequently than usual, during a flight.

7 Epileptic attacks become more likely.

8 Confusion may be precipitated in vulnerable patients by reduced oxygen levels, dehydration, anxiety and 'jet-lag'.

Advice to passengers

1 Always advise the airline of medical problems so that special arrangements can be made, e.g. extra oxygen, extra space, mobility aids, special diets.

2 Cabin crew are *not* nurses—special staff may need to be employed.

3 Airlines retain the right to refuse to transport passengers they consider unsuitable.

Further reading

Katoria M.S. (ed.) (1985) *Fits Faints and Falls in Old Age*. MTP Press, Lancaster.

Radebaugh T.S. (ed.), Hadley E. & Suzman R. (1985) In: *Clinics in Geriatric Medicine*. W.B. Saunders, London.

Chapter 9
Locomotor Disease

Bones

Ageing changes

Bone is a dynamic tissue which is being replaced and remodelled throughout life. The necessary equilibrium between bone production and resorption becomes unbalanced in later life. The result is a gradual and progressive loss of bone after the age of 35 years. This process affects trabecular bone more than cortical bone. However, the total bone mass becomes reduced but the nature of the bone remains normal. This natural and universal process results in osteoporosis. Bone loss is normally 0.2 per cent of total bone mass per year after the age of 35 years, rising to 1 per cent per annum in postmenopausal women.

In addition the shape of long bones alters with increasing age—the internal cavity increases in diameter and the outer cortical layer becomes thinner. The total bone diameter becomes expanded—the changes result in weaker bones.

Factors which potentiate osteoporosis

1 Failure to achieve maximal bone mass during adolescence and early adulthood.
2 Hormonal changes at the time of the menopause.
3 Longevity provides longer period for bone loss.
4 Poor calcium intake.
5 Inactivity—stressing of bones leads to strengthening.
6 Drug treatment, especially steroids.
7 Poor nutrition, including post-gastrectomy patients and those with malabsorption.
8 Genotype—family history—tall, slender, fair persons are most at risk.
9 Endocrine disorders, e.g. thyrotoxicosis, Cushing's disease, hyperparathyroidism and hypopituitarism.

Clinical osteoporosis

This is predominantly a female problem due to:
(i) Lower maximum bone development.
(ii) Effects of the menopause.
(iii) Prolonged life expectancy, i.e. a prolonged period of bone loss.

Symptoms

These only occur as a consequence of bone damage:
(i) Pain, due to fracture, e.g. of long bone or crush fracture of vertebral body.
(ii) Deformity—kyphosis (dowager's hump) due to vertebral collapse leads to shortening with reduction in crown to pubis measurement.

Investigations

X-rays (see Table 9.1):
(i) Thinning of bone texture when more than 30 per cent of bone mass is lost.
(ii) Presence of fractures, especially multiple vertebral deformity due to collapse of trabecular bone.

Biochemistry—normal but alkaline phosphatase may be raised during a period of active bone damage.

Table 9.1. Radiological evidence of vertebral crush fracture

255 per cent of women over 60 years
45 per cent of women over 80 years
25 per cent of men over 80 years

Complications of osteoporosis

(a) Fractures
(i) Crush fracture of vertebral bodies is most common and causes pain.
(ii) Colles fracture of distal end of radius affects 5 per cent of women aged 60 rising to 15 per cent aged 80. Lightweight splinting will minimize disability during healing. Unfortunately persistent disability after healing is common, irrespective of period of immobilization.

(iii) Neck of femur—rising incidence with increasing age (see Table 9.2). Incidence also greater than expected from demographic changes.

Table 9.2. Fracture neck of femur—Cambridge health district rate/1000 population in same age group

Age/years	Rate
−50	0.04
50–54	0.12
55–59	0.35
60–64	0.56
65–69	0.88
70–74	1.74
75–79	4.88
80–84	9.42
85–89	18.4
90–94	20.0
95+	25.0

(b) Use of resources
Fracture in osteoporotic bones now represents the third greatest cause for bed occupation in the NHS (in non-psychiatric hospitals). The cost of treatment of these patients is now more than one million pounds per week.

(c) Death
As a consequence of injury.

Prevention
(i) Maintain and encourage good nutrition, especially calcium intake of at least 1500 mg per day.
(ii) Hormone replacement—but at a physiological level only. No consensus view regarding duration of treatment or potential side effects or acceptability to patients; cyclical treatment recommended.
(iii) Fluoride supplements may strengthen bone.
(iv) Vitamin D supplements—beware the risk of hypercalcaemia.
(v) Diphosphonates—information from prolonged follow-up not yet available.
(vi) Calcitonin—inconvenient.

(vii) 'Blunderbuss treatment'—i.e. calcium, fluoride, vitamin D and oestrogens; some evidence that such polypharmacy may be an effective preventive measure.

(viii) Regular exercise within limitations; severe and excessive régimes may be counter-productive.

Treatment

(i) Identify and correct precipitating causes, e.g. steroid excess, thyrotoxicosis, hyperparathyroidism; this will prevent the situation getting worse, but does not return the bone to normal.

(ii) Analgesia for acute episodes of pain, usually severe backache. Can be stopped after spontaneous healing and repair although degenerative changes may still require symptomatic relief.

(iii) Encourage healing of fracture with immobilization but keep to a minimum if patient is frail or disabled from any other cause.

(iv) Repair fracture with internal fixation, encourage early remobilization; treatment of choice in lower limb fracture.

Osteomalacia

Defective calcification of bone due to vitamin D deficiency. The quantity of bone remains normal but the presence of uncalcified osteoid tissue leads to softening and weakness of the bony structure. Incidence—uncertain and depends on population studied.

(i) Admissions to Scottish departments of geriatric medicine 4 per cent.

(ii) Post-mortem study of elderly patients 12 per cent.

(iii) Biopsies on fractured neck of femur patients 25 per cent.

Causes

1 Reduced vitamin D availability

(i) Deficient diet, but diet is a poor source of vitamin D at all ages.

(ii) Lack of sunlight—endogenous production of vitamin D in skin on exposure to ultraviolet light is a prime source of vitamin D in all ages.

(iii) Malabsorption, e.g. coeliac disease, small bowel diverticular disease and postgastrectomy.

2 Impaired vitamin D metabolism
(i) Drug induced hepatic enzyme induction e.g. by anti-convulsants.
(ii) Renal failure impairs metabolism.

Symptoms and signs
(i) Pain, especially backache and limb girdle.
(ii) Muscular weakness and tenderness—a proximal myopathy is part of the clinical picture.
(iii) Fractures—because of bone fragility.
(iv) Impaired mobility, a waddling gait due to combination of pain and muscle weakness, rising from chairs and stair climbing particularly difficult.
(v) Presence of possible underlying causes, e.g. previous gastrectomy, known malabsorption or long history of anti-convulsant therapy and being housebound.

Investigations
(i) X-rays, only helpful in the rare event of a pseudo-fracture being demonstrated; bones are generally of low density but indistinguishable from osteoporosis.
(ii) Biochemical investigations—raised alkaline phosphatase, low calcium, low PO_4; it is unusual for all biochemical abnormalities to be present—sometimes all are absent. Serum vitamin D levels—not all low levels indicate the presence of osteomalacia.
(iii) Bone scan with radioactive-technetium-labelled diphosphate; osteomalacia picture—increased uptake in long bones and isolated 'hot spots'. Malignant deposits and Paget's disease also cause 'hot spots' but X-rays of these areas are usually characteristic.
(iv) Bone biopsy, the 'gold standard', taken from iliac crest; inconvenient and causes discomfort to the patient.

Treatment
1 If reduced availability of vitamin D, give oral vitamin supplements, e.g. combined calcium and vitamin D tablets.
2 If impaired metabolism, give Vitamin D metabolite (hydroxy-cholecalciferol).
NB Beware of hypercalcaemia as a complication of treatment.

Paget's disease of the bone

An imbalance between bone resorption and replacement. Osteoclastic activity is excessive and osteoblastic compensation attempts to repair the damage. Bone turnover may be increased to 20 times normal and the affected bone becomes distorted and weakened. The replacement bone is coarse fibred and disorganized and may affect single bone (10 per cent of cases) or several, mainly skull, spine and pelvis.

Incidence
Commonest in the UK, USA, Australasia, Germany and France. Rare in Scandinavia, the Middle and Far East and Africa. Its incidence rises with increasing age (see Table 9.3).

Table 9.3. Radiological and post-mortem incidence of Paget's disease of bone

Age	X-ray diagnosis (%)	Post-mortem diagnosis (%)
45–54	0.4	1.5
55–64	2.2	4.3
65–74	5.6	3.3
75–84	5.4	5.8
85+	9.1	11.1

Aetiology
Unknown, may be infective due to slow virus and is a potentially pre-malignant condition.

Symptoms and signs
1 Mainly asymptomatic—chance finding on X-ray or unexpected biochemical abnormality (raised alkaline phosphatase).
2 Deformity, e.g. skull, bowing of femora and tibiae.
3 Pain—localized or due to nerve entrapment.

Complications
1 Secondary osteoarthritis in adjacent joints.
2 Fracture of abnormal bone.

3 Nerve entrapment—deafness, paraplegia, hydrocephalus.
4 Malignant change.
5 Congestive cardiac failure.

Investigations
1 X-ray—distorted bone architecture and expanded bone.
2 Biochemistry—raised alkaline phosphatase and increased urinary hydroxyproline indicate active disease.
3 Bone scan—increased isotope uptake in affected bones.

Treatment
1 Nil if asymptomatic.
2 Analgesia if painful.
3 Calcitonin if pain resistant to simple analgesics and if there is evidence of pressure symptoms (inconvenient parenteral administration and expensive).
4 Diphosphonates—convenient oral treatment but may increase bone fragility.

Hyperparathyroidism

Primary hyperparathyroidism is said to have an incidence of 250 cases per million population per year—55 per cent of these cases will be in women over 70 years of age. The majority of these elderly patients will be asymptomatic and have been discovered on routine biochemical testing. Such patients should simply be observed and their biochemistry monitored. However, one-eighth of cases with a raised calcium level will have had documented episodes of confusion and dehydration and will merit treatment if otherwise well.

Confirmation of the diagnosis is difficult; a raised parathyroid hormone level should be sought. The abnormal glands must be identified before surgery by arteriography and ultrasound examination of the neck. In patients unable or unwilling to undergo surgery, treatment may be attempted with buffered phosphate.

Of the other causes of hypercalcaemia in old age that secondary to malignant disease is likely to cause most diagnostic difficulties. The hypercalcaemia of malignancy may respond to steroid treatment but that of hyperparathyroidism will not.

Joints

To many people joint problems seem to be part of growing older—arthritis is not universal and in old age it must be as precisely diagnosed as possible in order that appropriate treatment and management may be instigated.

	Patient consulting rate per 1000 persons (by age)					
	all ages	0–14	15–44	45–64	65–74	75+
Arthropathies	34	2	14	62	105	114

Osteoarthritis

1 Three-quarters of people over the age of 65 years have some X-ray evidence of osteoarthritis.

2 Two-thirds of people over 65 years have symptoms from osteoarthritis.

3 Aetiology usually unknown, i.e. primary osteoarthritis.

4 May be secondary to:

(i) Trauma leading to articular deformity.

(ii) Inflammatory disease, including gout and rheumatoid arthritis.

(iii) Aseptic necrosis.

(iv) Endocrine disease, e.g. myxoedema and acromegaly.

(v) Neuropathic, e.g. diabetic.

(vi) Hereditary disease, e.g. haemophilia.

(vii) Metabolic disease, e.g. Wilson's disease haemochromatosis.

5 Longstanding, complicated and burnt-out rheumatoid arthritis may be difficult to differentiate from generalized osteoarthritis in old age (see Table 9.4).

Table 9.4

Burnt-out rheumatoid arthritis	Generalized osteoarthritis
Bone erosions	Osteophytes
Osteoporosis	New bone formation
	Osteosclerosis

Osteoarthritis as a trigger to increasing immobility

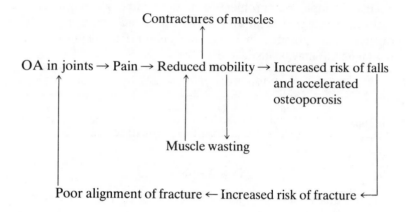

Treatment
1 Drugs
   (i) Simple analgesics if sufficient.
   (ii) Non-steroidal anti-inflammatory drugs if (i) is ineffective.
   (iii) Intra-articular injection of steroids, value debated, but sometimes worth trying if single joint is very disabling.
2 Physiotherapy—to strengthen muscles around affected joints.
3 Weight reduction to relieve strain on joints.
4 Aids
   (i) Stick or frame to spread weight and relieve damaged joints.
   (ii) Aids to overcome handicap, e.g 'helping hand' to overcome difficulty in bending to pick up objects from floor; 'stocking aid' to overcome inability to pull on stockings due to stiff back and hips; raised toilet seat and heel raised for shortened leg.
5 Rehouse—to avoid steps and stairs, etc.
6 Surgery—joint replacement.

The ideal patient for joint replacement
1 Refractory pain in single joint or only one severely affected joint.
2 Physically fit.
3 Mentally alert, orientated and well motivated.
4 Well nourished but not obese.

5 Unlikely to place unreasonable demands on new hip—i.e. normal mobility anticipated post-operatively and not excessive activity.

6 Of sufficient age so that patient is unlikely to outlive the new joint, i.e. aged 70+.

Complications of joint replacement

1 Infection—gallium scan may confirm—usually an early complication but may arise during any intercurrent infection.

2 Loosening of prosthesis—X-ray or bone scan may demonstrate.

3 Fracture of adjacent bone—visible on X-ray.

4 Patient outlives prosthesis and second operation needed.

5 Increased mobility reveals another pathology, e.g. angina results from the increased activity.

Rheumatoid arthritis

1 Inactive disease—an episode in earlier life which has burnt itself out but leaving many deformities and disabilities, sometimes progressing to a mixture of old rheumatoid arthritis and more recent osteoarthritis. Treatment as for osteoarthritis (see above).

2 Active disease—arising in old age for the first time or an exacerbation of old disease.

Active disease

1 May have very sudden and severe onset in old age.

2 May be self-limiting.

3 Equal sex incidence (females no longer predominate).

4 Less systemic complications.

5 Treatment may be more hazardous in old age.

Potential problems in the treatment of rheumatoid arthritis in elderly patients

1 Bed rest—if prolonged may make eventual remobilization impossible. Therefore tendency to keep rest to a minimum and concentrate on symptom relief and early mobilization.

2 Splinting—if bulky and heavy may significantly interfere with frail person's ability to maintain personal independence, especially if patient also has other disabilities. Night splints are acceptable to some patients. In very old patients the ability to move now is paramount—but the prevention of fixed flexion of the knees should be attempted if at all possible.

3 Rehabilitation—the presence of severe upper limb problems and other disorders, e.g. ischaemic heart disease, old stroke or amputation will significantly hinder a patient's ability to fully cooperate in an intensive physiotherapy programme, compromise may therefore be needed, and slow prolonged therapy may be more appropriate than short, sharp shock treatment.

4 Drugs—are often dangerous in old age, but important and valuable as:
(i) Quick symptom relief may be the best technique for preserving mobility and independence, therefore steroids (in spite of disadvantages) may be used earlier than in younger patients.

Gout	Pseudogout
Urate crystals	Pyrophosphate crystals
Usually the great toe affected	Usually the knee is affected
May be precipitated by:	No clear precipitation—but
1 Diuretics	acute illness or surgery may
2 Over-indulgence	be responsible
3 Fasting	
4 Excessive exercise or rest	
5 Acute illness or surgery	
Tophi may be present	Chondrocalcinosis may be present
Uric acid level raised	Uric acid may be normal
NSAIDs and specific treatment:	Anti-inflammatory treatment only
Colchicine	
Probenecid	
Allopurinol	
Erosion on X-ray	Chondrocalcinosis on X-ray
Obesity, increased blood pressure	Diabetes, hyperparathyroidism,
and ischaemic heart disease are	myxoedema are associated
associated conditions	conditions
Family history common	Family history less common

Fig. 9.1

(ii) Slow-acting antirheumatic drugs have effects generally too delayed for acceptable treatment in old age. Also increased risk of side effects because of age and pathological changes in other systems, e.g. renal impairment worsened by penicillamine and gold, visual impairment potentiated by chloroquine.

(iii) Non-steroidal anti-inflammatory drugs (NSAIDs)—main line treatment in active disease but all complications of treatment are more pronounced in the elderly, e.g. fluid retention, renal impairment and gastrointestinal bleeding.

Crystal arthropathy

Sudden severe pain causing immobility due to acute inflammatory response. All causes are age-related and sex incidence in old age approaches equality (see Fig. 9.1).

NB   Both conditions may be confused with acute joint sepsis. Aspiration for pus and crystals is the best technique for differentiation.

Infective arthropathy

1 To be considered when single joint is painful.

2 Difficult to diagnose in presence of old joint deformities.

3 May be confused with gout or pseudogout.

4 Systemic toxic effects may be minimal in the elderly.

5 Concurrent treatment may mask the problem, e.g. steroids, analgesics and antibiotics.

6 Aspirate if in doubt.

Muscle pain

Polymyalgia rheumatica

Generalized muscle pain and tenderness. Probably due to an arteritis and linked with giant cell arteritis—characterized by giant cells and granulomata found in the internal elastic lamina of the median layer of the artery plus narrowing of the lumen and generalized inflammatory changes in all layers of the vessel.

Cause—usually idiopathic but may be triggered by a viral infection or may indicate the presence of an underlying malignancy.

Diagnostic criteria
1 Bilateral shoulder pain and/or neck stiffness.
2 Onset of illness of less than 2 weeks, i.e. seek medical help within 2 weeks.
3 Initial ESR greater than 40.
4 Duration of morning stiffness of more than 1 hour.
5 Age greater than 65 years.
6 Depression and/or weight loss.
7 Bilateral tenderness in upper arms.

   Three positives = polymyalgia rheumatica. One positive+ abnormal temporal artery biopsy = polymyalgia rheumatica/giant cell arteritis. A successful therapeutic trial with steroids will confirm diagnosis—the response must be dramatic.
NB   Creatinine phosphokinase, muscle biopsy and EMG are all usually normal.

Complications of untreated polymyalgia rheumatica
1 Chronic disability.
2 Normochromic anaemia.
3 Hepatitis with raised alkaline phosphatase.
4 Progression to giant cell arteritis with major vessel occlusion, leading to blindness, stroke or myocardial infarction.

Treatment
1 Steroids 10–40 mg of prednisolone daily depending on severity of symptoms and threat of vessel occlusion. Overnight improvement in symptoms helps to confirm the diagnosis.
2 Dosage should be monitored according to symptoms and elevation of ESR.
3 Treatment may be necessary for 2 years or more and disease may recur and require more steroids.
4 Non-steroidal anti-inflammatory drugs (NSAIDs) may relieve symptoms but will not protect the patient from vascular occlusion.

Muscle weakness

Ageing changes
Muscle bulk and effectiveness decline with increasing age. Musculature becomes atrophic and paler in colour due to a decrease in muscle fibres, an increase in fat and fibrous tissue and increased

deposition of lipochrome pigment. These changes may not be exclusively due to ageing but may merely reflect the more sedentary life in old age in developed countries—muscle bulk can still be increased in the elderly by regular exercise. Neuronal impairment may be another explanation for the 'ageing changes'.

Muscle pathology in old age

1 Myositis
Tender and weak muscles
Rarely infective in old age, but transient post-viral symptoms are common
Often associated with underlying malignancy
Often associated with skin involvement—dermatomyositis

2 Myopathy
Weak muscles usually proximal and without tenderness
Non-metastatic complication of malignancy commonest group
Endocrine—Cushings
          Thyrotoxicosis
          Diabetes mellitus—amyotrophy
Drug induced, e.g. steroids and alcohol
Metabolic, usually due to hypokalaemia (endocrine or drug induced)
Also vitamin D deficiency (part of osteomalacia)

3 Myasthenia
Exaggerated fatiguability; ten per cent of all cases occur in old age
Idiopathic—corrected by Tensilon
May be associated with underlying malignancy—poor response to Tensilon
May be drug induced (Penicillamine and aminoglycosides)

Investigation of muscle disease
1 Raised creatinine phosphokinase indicates muscle damage.
2 EMG helps differentiate neurogenic and primary muscle disorders.
3 Biopsy—difficult and requires skilled and experienced interpretation, therefore best results from specialized centres.
4 Tensilon test—in suspected myasthenia.

5 Specific tests to confirm underlying cause, e.g. thyroid function tests.

Treatment

1 Correct precipitating cause, if possible.
2 Anticholinesterases in myasthenia.
3 Steroids worth trying in malignant myopathy, especially polymyositis/dermatomyositis but beware of causing steroid myopathy.

Further reading

Wright V. (ed.) (1983) *Bone Disease in the Elderly.* Churchill Livingstone, Edinburgh.

Chapter 10
Cerebrovascular Disease

The incidence of cerebrovascular disease and completed stroke rises steeply with age and constitutes the third most common cause of death after heart disease and cancer (see Fig. 10.1). Two-thirds of all male and almost 90 per cent of female victims are aged 65 years and over. Interruption of blood flow may be due to both intra- and extra-cerebral causes.

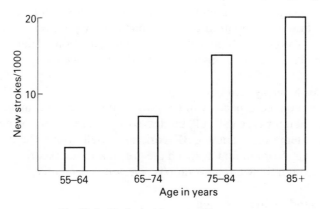

Fig. 10.1. Stroke incidence at different ages.

Cerebral blood flow (CBF)

1 Diminishes progressively with age, as does cerebral glucose metabolism.
2 Has a bigger range of variability in the elderly.
3 In the young is kept constant despite large and sometimes abrupt changes in arterial, venous and intracranial pressures by a mechanism of autoregulation which is commonly defective in the elderly.

Cerebral autoregulatory mechanisms

1 Myogenic reflex response of smooth muscle in cerebral vessels.
2 Response of smooth muscle to metabolic changes, especially pH, PCO_2 and PO_2.
3 Autonomic nervous system (ANS) reflexes.

Cerebral blood flow: effects of ageing and disease

Healthy old people
CBF is maintained but at lower level. It rises in the relevant cortical area with physical and mental activity, falls to low levels in slow wave sleep but rises again in rapid eye movement (REM) sleep. This phase is less prominent in the elderly and is further suppressed by psychosedative drugs.

Arterial oxygen tension
Hypoxia causes increased tissue levels of lactic acid with increased blood flow but impaired cerebral function. A progressive fall in arterial oxygen tension will cause increasing brain failure and eventual loss of consciousness despite the increased CBF.

Chronic brain syndromes
CBF is reduced especially in the grey matter in senile dementia of the Alzheimer type (SDAT) but less so and more patchily in multi-infarct dementia. Total CBF correlates well with mental performance. Normal flow through the grey matter markedly exceeds that through the white; this ratio is reversed in dementia.

Longstanding hypertension
Cerebral autoregulation shifts to a higher level. Abrupt lowering of blood pressure (BP) causes a fall in perfusion. Slow, gradual reduction is well tolerated and autoregulation resets at a lower, more normal level.

Acute stroke
Perfusion is much reduced or absent at the site of the infarct. Surrounding hyperaemia or 'luxury perfusion' occurs due to tissue acidosis. The autoregulatory mechanism may be out of action for several days and the brain is especially at risk from high or low blood pressure at this time.

Transient cerebral ischaemic attacks
Disturbances of CBF and autoregulation persist for hours after an attack and some disturbance of flow may remain for weeks. In carotid artery disease or vertebral artery disease flow in the appropriate territory is reduced.

Normal pressure hydrocephalus
CBF is reduced in keeping with the size of the ventricles (see Chapter 11).

Cerebrovascular disease

This may present in a variety of ways:
1 Transient ischaemic attack (TIA).
2 Reversible ischaemic neurological deficit (RIND).
3 Stroke.
4 Multi-infarct dementia.
5 Pseudobulbar palsy and walking difficulties.
6 Epilepsy.
7 Pseudo-Parkinsonism.
The main risk factors are:
1 *Hypertension*—increased risk at all ages for both haemorrhagic and non-haemorrhagic stroke.
2 *Cardiac disease*—estimated 15 per cent of strokes due to cardiac embolism; atrial fibrillation has a 30 per cent incidence of TIA or stroke.
3 *Metabolic*—especially diabetes mellitus and hyperlipidaemia.
4 *Cigarette smoking.*
5 *Hypotension*—due to disease or drugs in the presence of narrowed intra- and extracranial arteries and impaired cerebral vascular autoregulation.
6 *Increased blood viscosity*—even high normal haematocrit is a risk factor for stroke.
Atheroma of major intra- and extracranial arteries is the most common underlying cause, but the role of cardiac disease is increasingly recognized. The atheromatous lesions which give rise to stenosis and embolism are patchy and their location critical. Since the 'villain of the piece' (atheroma) has been building up for many years, even from childhood, prevention is to be attempted in the young and middle-aged. Prevention of clinical manifestations can

be attempted at any age by management of the known risk factors listed above.

Transient cerebral ischaemic attacks (TIAs)

1 Transient cerebral ischaemic attacks (TIAs) are focal episodes, usually repeated, of a sensory or motor impairment due to temporary inadequacy of blood flow to a localized area of the brain. Each attack lasts usually just a few minutes, occasionally much longer but, by definition, not more than 24 hours. They leave no residual signs. It is useful to consider them in terms of the main vascular supply because the presentation and prognosis often differs.

2 In cases with a disturbance in the territory of the carotid artery the clinical features may include:

- Hemiparesis, hemisensory disturbance, dysphasia, hemianopia.
- Monocular blindness (*amaurosis fugax*).
- A carotid artery bruit heard in the neck.

3 In vertebro-basilar ischaemic episodes there can be more difficulty in assessing the clinical significance of the presenting features, which may include:

- Vertigo, nystagmus, ataxia.
- Facial paraesthesiae, especially perioral.
- Visual field loss, 'flashing lights' or diplopia.
- Dysarthia, dysphagia.
- Weakness or numbness which may be unilateral or bilateral.
- Global amnesia.

4 Despite the protean manifestations of TIA it is important to remember that not all episodes of impaired cerebration with amnesia, dizziness, unsteadiness and so forth can be attributed to this cause. A rigorous search must be made (see also Chapter 8).

5 Recurrent attacks of TIA are usually territory specific on account of intravascular laminar flow or 'streaming' which reduces the scatter of emboli and because of critical 'watershed' areas between different arterial supplies.

Reversible ischaemic neurological deficit (RIND)

A reversible ischaemic neurological deficit is as for a TIA but with a duration of over 24 hours up to 3 weeks.

Prognosis

Transient cerebral ischaemic attacks may cease, persist or proceed to a stroke in about equal proportions; most die from heart disease. The extra risk of stroke is maximal in the early days or weeks after the initial attack. Attacks in the vertebrobasilar territory are more likely to be recurrent but are uncommonly followed by a stroke. The opposite obtains in the territory of the internal carotid artery. Stroke tends to affect the same area as for the preceding TIA. The risk of stroke is highest in hypertensives. After 6 months, free from TIA, the risk is as for age and sex together with other known risk factors.

Management of TIA

1 The cause must be sought and treated (see above). Highly specialized or invasive investigations, e.g. angiography are rarely required except in the 'young old' when surgery is contemplated.

2 Even if carotid stenosis is proven, it is not known if endarterectomy provides worthwhile treatment; also there is no clear indication for external carotid/internal carotid bypass operation.

3 Aspirin is the best choice for antiplatelet activity. Quite low doses appear to be effective, e.g 75 mg daily. We do not routinely use anticoagulants, sulphinpyrazone or dipyridamole for TIA.

4 For crescendo TIAs a heparin infusion is given until the attacks cease followed by warfarin for 6 months. If TIAs are infrequent we use aspirin from the start.

5 A soft collar may help by limiting neck movement in cervical spondylosis.

The completed stroke

An enduring neurological defect due to cerebrovascular disease. About 80 per cent of first-ever strokes are due to cerebral infarction, about 15 per cent due to primary intracerebral haemorrhage and the remainder due to subarachnoid haemorrhage. The commonest clinical picture is hemiplegia but almost any combination of neurological signs or symptoms may be due to stroke, especially:

• Impairment of consciousness.

• Flaccidity, spasticity, dysarthria, dysphagia (usually temporary).

• Loss of sensation and awareness in the affected limbs.

• Dysphasia (dominant hemisphere), agnosia (non-dominant hemisphere).

- Urinary incontinence (usually temporary).
- Intellectual failure.
- Hemianopia.
- Emotional disturbance—anxiety, depression.

Textbooks of neurology or medicine should be consulted for descriptions of the various clinical pictures. The diagnosis is usually obvious but attention should be paid to the following:

1 Likely underlying pathology, to give guidance with respect to treatment and prognosis, e.g. embolism or the rare case due to giant cell arteritis.

2 Documentation of the extent of the neurological deficit and functional impairment.

3 Other aspects of the patient's physical and mental state prior and subsequent to the stroke, e.g. personality and ability to cope.

4 Unusual presentations which may be perplexing. These are frequently due to small discrete lesions for example:

(a) Apraxia, agnosia and spatial disorientation with no sensory or motor loss or mental confusion—lesion in non-dominant parietal lobe rearward of the post-central gyrus.

(b) Isolated hemianopia—lesion in occipital lobe (macula may be spared).

(c) Diplopia, vertigo, dysarthria and ataxia with or without other cranial nerve palsies or long tract signs in various combinations—lesion of the brainstem.

(d) Language difficulty without hemiplegia—lesion in dominant temporal lobe.

(e) Isolated sensory loss in limbs(s)—lesion of sensory cortex.

5 Severe receptive dysphasia and the fluent type of expressive dysphasia may mimic confusion or dementia.

6 Emotional disturbance:

(a) Uncontrollable weeping or agression—left cerebral lesion.

(b) Apathy with denial or minimalization—right cerebral lesion.

Differential diagnosis

1 Causes of loss of consciousness:

(a) Brain damage—vascular, traumatic or infective, e.g. meningitis or encephalitis.

(b) Intact brain—affected by drugs or abnormal metabolism, e.g. hypoglycaemia, myxoedema.

2 Causes of hemiplegia:

(a) Subdural haematoma, trauma may be trivial.

(b) Neoplasm, occasionally presents acutely.

(c) Post-epileptic (Todd's) paralysis, resolves spontaneously in minutes, hours, rarely days.

(d) Hypoglycaemia, an uncommon but treatable cause.

Prognosis

Prognosis for recovery depends upon the size and location of the lesion and upon the associated pathology. Most deeply comatose patients die within hours or days, most mentally alert patients survive the acute phase unless the lesion progresses. Functional recovery is adversely affected by:

- Severity of stroke including loss of intellect.
- Paralysis of conjugate ocular gaze.
- Homonymous hemianopia.
- Sensory neglect, apraxia, motor perseveration.
- Intractable depression, dementia.
- Persistent incontinence.
- Negative attitudes of carers.

Useful recovery may still take place even after 6 months and it can be difficult to foresee the outcome before about 3 months.

Investigation of stroke

The great majority of strokes are due to infarct, and in about a third there is antecedent hypotension as a precipitant—sleep, drugs, gastrointestinal bleeding, myocardial infarction or pulmonary infarction.

Detailed investigation is not necessary in every case, although it is helpful to know the nature of the brain lesion and why it occurred. Also it is necessary to know the associated pathology and to decide what can and should be treated. Mostly these decisions are made on the basis of the clinical history and physical examination supported by the investigations common to newly admitted patients, viz. routine blood, urine, ECG, chest X-ray. More specialized investigations are required to provide extra information in selected cases.

Consider:

(a) Skull X-ray—?calcification of tumour, shift of mid-line structure, fractures.

(b) CT scan—differentiates cerebral haemorrhage from infarct and detects other pathology such as subdural haematoma or tumour.

(c) Radionuclide imaging—altered perfusion demonstrable within hours.

(d) Lumbar puncture—rarely justified and is hazardous if IC pressure is raised; only if meningitis or subarachnoid haemorrhage is suspected

(e) EEG—if epilepsy is suspected.

(f) 24-hour ECG—to detect episodes of arrhythmia.

Management of stroke

In the acute phase much medical and nursing support may be required to manage the unconscious or mentally obtunded patient. It is not yet clear whether the patient is generally better off in hospital or at home. Interpretation of published data is difficult. The worst cases tend to be admitted to general wards, the specialist stroke units being more selective. For a given level of initial disability, family attitudes and responses are major determinants of functional ability in the months and years following a stroke. In our practice we focus our main rehabilitative effort on the middle grade of disability and less on the 'hopeless' or the mild cases.

Reasons for admission to hospital

1 Damage limitation—by maintenance of airway, blood pressure and hydration.

2 Prevention and treatment of complications.

3 To ascertain and treat the cause, e.g. metabolic change, giant cell arteritis, factors producing hypotension.

4 To confirm the diagnosis—?ischaemic infarct or haemorrhage; exclude subdural haematoma, neoplasm, meningitis.

5 Rehabilitation.

6 Lack of family and domiciliary support services at home.

The last mentioned is much the most common reason for British general practitioners requesting admission. Given good home circumstances and domiciliary support which can be mobilized rapidly, even severe strokes can be managed at home. In most cases diagnostic uncertainty (the second commonest reason for admission) could be resolved by the availability of a rapid domiciliary and outpatient diagnostic service. Because of the risk of converting an ischaemic to an haemorrhagic infarct the use of anticoagulants in the acute stage of cerebral embolism is controversial. The previous recommendation was to wait 3 weeks to allow the infarct to heal but the risk of recurrent embolism is high (40 per cent), and a further stroke may occur early. Hence the interest in early anticoagulation with heparin followed by warfarin, provided there is no evidence of bleeding on CT scan or LP. Long-term warfarin is indicated if the risk of embolism persists. In the very old and disabled there are often practical problems and medical contraindications to this line of treatment and our practice tends to be conservative.

Complications: avoidance and treatment

1 Retention or incontinence of urine or faeces

- Sensitive, encouraging nursing; may need temporary appliance (male). Catheter best avoided but valuable if prolonged loss of consciousness and is essential for retention; examine the rectum initially and at intervals.
- Attention to both diuretics and dietetics, may need stool softeners and laxatives.

2 Deep vein thrombosis (DVT) and risk of pulmonary embolus

- DVT occurs in more than half of cases.
- Prevention by early mobilization, full hydration, TED stockings and low-dose heparin (hazards if intracerebral bleed); in general we do not give prophylactic anticoagulant.

3 Chest infection

- Commonly diagnosed when the real cause of respiratory distress is multiple small pulmonary emboli.
- Prophylactic physiotherapy.
- Appropriate antibiotic.
- Maintenance of airway and avoidance of inhalation of food.

4 Dysphagia

- Nasopharyngeal reflux and tracheal aspiration giving pneumonitis.
- Especially with brain stem lesion.
- May unmask lower oesophageal pathology.
- May need temporary naso-gastric tube.

5 Pressure sores
(see Chapter 19)

6 *Pain in paretic limbs*
• Very common, often multiple causes.
• Upper limb—consider capsulitis, subluxation, contracture, fracture.
• Lower limb—consider especially DVT.
• Both upper and lower, if none of the above, consider thalamic pain. Try anticonvulsant and or antidepressant.

7 *Spasticity*
• Should be preventable with appropriate positioning and physiotherapy techniques.
• Also treat cofactors of spasticity such as pain, anxiety, distended viscus.
• Trial of antispasticity drug, e.g. baclofen starting with a small dose and gradually increasing, often not well tolerated.

8 *Emotional disturbance*
• Mental depression may be profound, try antidepressants.
• Catastrophic and bereavement type reactions (see also Chapter 21). Time, emotional support and encouragement are a great help.
• Maximize involvement in self care as well as social activities.

Rehabilitation and prognosis
See Chapter 6 regarding rehabilitation and prognosis in stroke, especially Table 6.2.

Planning for return home
When there is considerable disability great care must be taken to make a realistic assessment of the capacity to cope both of the patient and the key supporting relatives. Particular attention should be paid to the following:
1 Key carer(s) to work with the patient and remedial therapists in the hospital so that all are aware of each other's capabilities and of the special 'handling' techniques required.
2 Home assessment visit with patient, therapist and key carer.
3 Attendance at day hospital twice or thrice weekly before and after discharge.
4 Appropriate adaptations to clothing and to facilities at home to simplify activities of daily living.
5 Review progress at day hospital and consider transfer to a day centre, stroke club or general purpose old people's club.

6 Keep in touch with the key supporters and offer respite care, as day case or inpatient.

7 When in doubt about discharge despite appropriate preparation let patient go home on trial basis. The patient's response to this is vital. Some most unlikely cases do very well!

8 Failure of patient and or key carer to adjust to the new situation spells long-term misery for all concerned. Support may be eroded by severe and persistent anxiety, guilt, overprotection and lack of realism. A stroke club is better than medical help with these problems.

Diffuse cerebrovascular disease; multi-infarct disease

Cerebrovascular disease may present as a diffuse, insidious and often stepwise chronic brain failure with increasing mental and physical disability. The risk factors are as for TIA and stroke and the main clinical features are listed in Table 10.1. The pathology is multiple cortical and subcortical infarcts of variable size rather than simply 'narrowing of the arteries'. Probably around 15 per cent of all dementias in the elderly are due to this cause (see Chapter 7). The recorded incidence will vary both with the population studied and the method of diagnosis. Parkinson's disease (PD) may be mimicked but rigidity is usually much more marked in the lower limbs and gives the impression of the patient actively resisting which is quite unlike PD. Also there is no response to levodopa unless the

Table 10.1. Clinical features of diffuse cerebrovascular disease

---

Mental
Intellectual failure—progressive
Personality changes—lack of drive, reduced spontaneity,poverty of movement
 —emotionally labile, cantankerous even paranoid behaviour
Physical
Recurrent TIA, RIND or little strokes
Bilateral pyramidal tract lesions—progressive
Disintegration of walking pattern—unsteady with broad base,'stammering' gait,
 tendency to fall backwards
Supranuclear bulbar (pseudobulbar) palsy
 —dysarthria
 —dysphagia
 —emotional incontinence
Epilepsy of late onset
Incontinence

---

two diseases coexist. Aspiration pneumonia is not uncommon in the more severe cases.

There can be walking apraxia and loss of posture control without much in the way of paresis or sensory loss. The patient tends to fall backwards, walks with a shuffling gait, repeatedly coming to a halt and starting again only with difficulty—the stammering Petren gait. The feet at times appear to 'glue' to the floor yet if a low obstruction is placed in front of the patient she is able to step over it! Leaning backwards and other quite bewildering gait and balance problems can occur even with little dementia. These cases tax the patience and ingenuity of us all!

Treatment is as for TIA and physiotherapy is valuable to stave off immobility for as long as possible. Drugs such as chlormethiazole, the phenothiazines and the butyrophenones are used for the control of the various mental disturbances (see Chapter 7).

Epilepsy

Epilepsy appearing for the first time in late life is most likely to be due to cerebrovascular disease but 15–20 per cent of cases will have an intracranial tumour and another 10 per cent Alzheimer's disease. A fit may herald a stroke especially a haemorrhage or be followed by transient hemiplegia; other presentations include:

• Bouts of mental confusion.
• Paroxysmal pain on the paretic side in a patient with stroke.
• Akinetic attacks—the patient suddenly crumples to the ground without loss of consciousness.

Apart from cerebrovascular disease, tumour and Alzheimer's disease consider:

• Cardiac arrhythmia.
• Drugs known to be epileptogenic, viz. phenothiazines, tricyclical antidepressives, corticosteroids.
• Hypoglycaemic episodes.
• Abrupt withdrawal of alcohol or psychosedative drug.
• Head injury.

If the attacks are frequent, standard anticonvulsant therapy is employed.

Further reading

Bamford J., Sandercock P., Warlow C. & Gray M. (1986) Why are patients with acute stroke admitted to hospital? *British Medical Journal*, **292**, 1369–72.

Dennis M.S. & Warlow C.P. (1987) Stroke: Incidence, risk factors and outcome. *British Journal of Hospital Medicine*, **37**, 194–8.

Isaacs B. (1985)The central nervous system—stroke. In: Brocklehurst J.C. (ed.) *Textbook of Geriatric Medicine and Gerontology*, 3rd ed., pp. 427–48. Churchill Livingstone, Edinburgh.

Tallis R.C. (1985) Acute stroke illness in the elderly. In: Lye M. *Acute Geriatric Medicine*, pp. 37–58. MTP Press, Lancaster.

Chapter 11
Other Diseases of the Central Nervous System

Clinical examination

Age changes alone will alter the clinical signs and symptoms to be expected (see Table 11.1). Apart from the main illness, multiple pathology is commonly present with, for example, pre-existing central nervous system (CNS) diseases as well as other pathology affecting the neuromuscular system such as diabetes mellitus or rheumatoid arthritis. Higher cerebral functions must not be neglected. Elderly patients often have small pupils and it is not possible to obtain a good view with the ophthalmoscope without mydriasis. The important macular area and fovea is particularly difficult to visualize (see also Chapter 19).

Table 11.1. Neurological norms in the elderly

The following 'abnormal' clinical signs are not uncommonly found and may be of little or no diagnostic importance in the individual patient:
- Primitive reflexes such as the palmomental and the glabellar tap.
- Small slowly reacting pupils.
- Muscle wasting, especially the small muscles of the hands.
- Isolated fasciculation, especially in the calves.

Impairment of:
- Recent memory (benign senescent forgetfulness) and flexibility of intellect (see Chapter 7).
- Special senses (see Chapter 19).
- Posture control with increased angle of sway (see Chapter 8).

Reduction or absence of:
- Upward gaze.
- Jaw jerk.
- Corneal reflex.
- Ankle jerks (see Chapter 5).
- Vibration sense at the ankle.
- Two point discrimination.
- Perception of modest temperature change—ambient or local to skin surface.

Table 11.2 gives a guide to specific neurological investigations but these should be discussed with the appropriate specialist to

Table 11.2. A guide to neurological investigations

X-ray skull:
Looking for suspected:
    Fracture
    Midline shift
    Bone lesion—erosion, metastases or Paget's disease
    Enlargement of auditory canal or pituitary fossa
    Calcified tumour or aneurysm

X-ray spine:
    Root entrapment
    Cord compression

Computerized tomography (CT):
    Head injury—contusion or haematoma
    Cerebral/cerebellar infarction or haemorrhage
    Cerebral tumour or abscess
    Subdural haematoma, subarachnoid haemorrhage
    Normal-pressure hydrocephalus, cortical atrophy
    Cord compression or root entrapment (if whole body scanner available)

Radionuclide imaging (RNI):
    Cerebral tumour or abscess
    Chronic subdural haematoma
    Cerebral infarction—CT better if available (low density area within 48 hours)
    Encephalitis
    Perfusion studies

Lumbar puncture:
    Meningism, e.g. meningitis, encephalitis, subarachnoid haemorrhage
    Cord compression (for contrast studies)
    Acute post-infection polyneuropathy, multiple sclerosis, neurosyphilis

Angiography:
    Rarely in the elderly
    Thromboembolism, carotid stenosis
    Intracranial aneurysm

EEG occasionally in:
    Epilepsy
    Focal hemisphere lesion

Electrophysiological studies:
    Peripheral and entrapment neuropathies
    Motor neurone disease
    Primary disorder of muscle (biopsy may be needed)

---

clarify both the discriminative value of the proposed investigation as well as the requisite degree of patient cooperation.

Parkinson's disease and other Parkinsonian syndromes

Parkinson's disease (PD) or paralysis agitans is an incurable, progressive, degenerative disease characterized clinically by the development of two or more of the following features:
- Bradykinesia.
- Rigidity.
- Resting tremor, 5/sec, worse on stress, ceasing in sleep.
- Impaired posture control.

Often augmented later by:
- Shuffling or festinant (hurrying) gait and falls.
- Unblinking, expressionless ('reptilian') face with widened palpebral fissures.
- Weight loss.
- Dysphonia, dysarthria, drooling and dysphagia.
- Mental depression.
- Heartburn and constipation.
- Micrographia.
- Intellectual failure.
- Muscle weakness and pain.

Cerebrovascular disease is not regarded as a cause of Parkinsonism but since Parkinson's disease is the commonest disease of the nervous system after cerebrovascular disease the two not uncommonly coexist and the clinical picture combines features of both disorders.

Prevalence
In a recent UK study the prevalence was estimated to be $254/10^5$ in the decade aged 60–69 rising to $1924/10^5$ in those over the age of 80 years. There is an ineluctable progression of disability over the years. Various rating scales are used to document this, e.g. Table 11.3.

Differential diagnosis of Parkinsonism
This term is used to describe a clinical picture, akin to PD but with significant differences in pathology. Dopamine–acetycholine

Table 11.3. Hoehn and Yahr rating scale for Parkinson's disease

Stage I	Unilateral involvement only, minimal or no functional impairment.
Stage II	Bilateral involvement, without impairment of balance.
Stage III	First sign of impaired righting reflexes. Unsteadiness as patient turns or when pushed from standing equilibrium. Functionally restricted but physically capable of leading an independent life; disability mild to moderate.
Stage IV	Fully developed, severely disabling disease; still able to walk and stand unassisted, but markedly incapacitated.
Stage V	Confined to bed or wheelchair unless aided.

(Source: *Neurology* 1967; **17**: 427–67.)

imbalance is common to all cases but the response to levodopa treatment varies enormously. This heterogeneous collection of disorders includes:

1 Idiopathic Parkinsonism
- Paralysis agitans (young patients).
- Late-onset Parkinsonism ('senile' type).
- Striatonigral degeneration (rare).

2 Symptomatic Parkinsonism
- Postencephalitic.
- Drug-induced, e.g. phenothiazines, butyrophenones.
- Toxic (e.g. MPTP, manganese).
- Trauma (e.g. boxers).

3 Multisystem disorders
- Progressive supranuclear palsy (Steele–Richardson–Olszewski syndrome).
- Shy–Drager syndrome.
- Senile dementia of the Alzheimer type (SDAT).

Parkinsonism of late life is a diagnostic minefield. Benign essential tremor is most often misinterpreted and the general slowing up of early Parkinsonism may be attributed to depression, arthritis or hypothyroidism. Furthermore, multiple pathology is commonly the setting for Parkinsonism especially mental depression, dementia and heart disease. The latter rarely precludes low-dose levodopa therapy. Antipsychotics, often (and very often unwisely) prescribed for elderly people may produce Parkinsonism.

Pathology

Most new cases of Parkinson's disease are of unknown aetiology although a slow virus is postulated. Postencephalitic cases are now extremely rare. The essential pathological features are:

- Loss of melanin-pigmented neurones in the substantia nigra.
- Presence of neuronal inclusion (Lewy) bodies.
- Progressive loss of dopamine neurotransmission leading to an increase in cholinergic transmission.
- Additional neurotransmitter imbalances affecting, e.g. noradrenaline, serotonin and gamma-aminobutyric acid.

Factors affecting drug therapy for Parkinsonism

A Older patients

1 Have more widespread brain disorder due to age, developing senile dementia of the Alzheimer type (SDAT) or other pathology.
2 Are more liable to adverse effects from anti-Parkinsonian therapy.
3 Are less able to respond satisfactorily and may not respond at all to exogenous dopamine on account of a variable degree of post-synaptic degeneration.

B Younger patients

Usually present with idiopathic PD in 'pure' form, have intact post-synaptic receptors and can expect a good response to dopamine.

C Patients with other syndromes

Usually have post-synaptic degeneration and cannot be expected to respond to exogenous dopamine, e.g. progressive supranuclear palsy and Shy–Drager syndrome.

D Multiple pathology

1 Presence of mental disorder (especially depression), heart disease and prostatism, must be taken into account.
2 SDAT may be part of the PD syndrome with selective impairment of visuospatial tasks making the total disability much worse than is evident solely from the severity of the motor disorder.

3 Autonomic degeneration may in part account for:
- Constipation, worsened by anticholinergics, not by levodopa.
- Drooling due to impaired facial, oropharyngeal and oesophageal motility.
- Periodic severe sweating ('sweating crises') but always consider infection.
- Bladder malfunction; prostatism and anticholinergics exacerbate this problem.
- Orthostatic hypotension (see also Chapter 12).

Treatment for Parkinsonism
1 Withdraw offending agent in drug-induced Parkinsonism. Slow recovery usually occurs.
2 Counselling with respect to long-term strategy. Put patient in contact with the Parkinson's Disease Society (address at end of chapter). Keep Moving! Advise against driving.
3 Remedial therapy including the use of aids to daily living beginning with the simplest devices such as a walking stick, Velcro fasteners for clothing and a board under the mattress to facilitate turning over in bed (see also Chapter 6).
4 Drug therapy. Avoid use of anticholinergics routinely because their benefits are outweighed by the disadvantages, especially acute confusion and toxic psychosis. Start with low dose levodopa in a preparation combined with sufficient peripheral decarboxylase inhibitor and cautiously increase at weekly intervals to a maintenance level; initially keeping well below the point at which benefit is marred by adverse effects.
5 65–75 per cent of patients experience worthwhile improvement with respect to bradykinesia and rigidity but not tremor. The progress of the disease is not prevented.
6 Most elderly patients manage satisfactorily on a total daily dose of between 100–400 mg levodopa daily in divided doses, 2–4 times in the day.
7 Marked fluctuations in response with episodes of peak dose dyskinesia and end of dose deterioration or 'freezing' are treated by spreading the dopamine dose more thinly throughout the 24 hours, say 6 doses daily. Also consider use of bromocriptine (a dopaminergic agonist) or selegiline (a monoamine oxidase B inhibitor) and thereby reduce the dose of levodopa. As the disease progresses fluctuations become increasingly unpredictable, the 'Yo-yo' or 'On-off' phenomenon.

8 The adverse effects of levodopa include, gastrointestinal upset, cardiac arthythmias, postural hypotension, involuntary movements, agitation, insomnia and toxic psychosis. Depression is a most important complication both of Parkinsonism and of levodopa therapy but it usually reponds to tricyclics.

Other disorders with involuntary movements

Drug-induced extrapyramidal disorders
See Table 11.4.

Essential tremor
1 A common disorder of unknown aetiology. The incidence increases with age; rarely a gross disability.
2 Fine or course rhythmical movement affecting head, face, tongue and limbs; severity increases slowly over time.
3 Benign, familial, dominant trait.
4 Present at rest, exaggerated by stress, and volitional movement, ceases in sleep.
5 No relationship to Parkinson's disease but is more common.
6 Often relieved by small amounts of alcohol (useful socially) but a beta–blocker is first choice, e.g. propranolol.

Intention tremor
1 Usually seen in multiple sclerosis and cerebellar disorders.
2 Comes on with movement, e.g. writing, buttoning clothes, not present at rest.
3 Can occur in isolation with no other physical signs and no drug treatment.
4 No specific medical treatment.

Progressive supranuclear palsy
Also referred to as the Richardson–Steele–Olszewski syndrome. A multisystem disorder which usually develops as an atypical extrapyramidal disorder and progresses more rapidly than PD. Possibly 5 per cent of patients initially diagnosed as PD eventually develop signs of it, especially:
1 Gait disturbance and falls with some memory and personality deterioration due to subcortical dementia.
2 Failure of voluntary eye movement particularly downward gaze.

Table 11.4. Drug-induced extrapyramidal disorders

	Parkinsonism	Dystonia	Akathisia	Tardive dyskinesia/orofacial dyskinesia
Clinical picture	Resembles PD but without the characteristic resting tremor	Acute dystonia, dysarthia, mutism, occulogyric crises	Compulsive psycho motor restlessness 'the jitters' plus anxiety; occasional early features of PD	Abnormal movements affecting especially the mouth, tongue and face. Resembles Huntington's chorea but without dementia
Drugs implicated	BPh, PTZ (DA blockers), reserpine (DA depleter), alphamethyl dopa (false neurotransmitter), MPTP (neurotoxicity)	PTZ especially trifluoperazine and fluphenazine. Also metoclopramide and levodopa	PTZ especially prochlorperazine and perphenazine	Virtually all effective antipsychotic drugs—PTZ, BPh and metoclopramide
Induction dose/period	Dose-related effect with PTZ over weeks or months. Occurs with conventional doses of BPH. Misuse of MPTP	Not dose-related, acute sensitivity reaction, early (24–48 hours) in treatment	Even small doses, over days or weeks	Usually large cumulative dose over many months or years; also occurs spontaneously in about 2% elderly people
Management	Reduce or withdraw offending drugs. Resolves in 3–12 months. Anticholinergics speed resolution, e.g. benztropine (orally). Avoid levodopa, it may increase psychosis. May be essential to keep the antipsychotic going despite the AE. The effect of MPTP is irreversible	Reduce or withdraw offending drugs. Rapidly abolished by anticholinergics e.g. iv benztropine	Reduce or withdraw offending drugs; try anticholinergics but response generally unsatisfactory	Reduce or withdraw offending drugs; usually slow improvement over months or years but may be permanent. PTZ persists in tissues for years
Likely victims	Elderly patients on long-term antipsychotic drugs	Young patients on short-term treatment	Elderly patients	Elderly females especially those with pre-existing brain damage

AE = adverse effect
PD = Parkinson's disease
BPh = butyrophenone(s)
MPTP = methylphenyltetrahydropyridine
PTZ = phenothiazine(s)
DA = dopamine

3 Severe axial rigidity sometimes with extended rather than flexed postures and pseudobulbar palsy.

4 There is no specific therapy; poor response to levodopa.

Shy–Drager syndrome

An uncommon multisystem disorder of late middle life with variable features of autonomic and extrapyramidal degeneration. Orthostatic hypotension is the main problem but there may also be loss of libido, nocturnal incontinence and anhidrosis. Management of the orthostatic hypotension includes:

1 Whole body head-up tilt at night to promote sodium retention.

2 Fludrocortisone in small doses to expand the extracellular fluid volume and enhance vascular reactivity.

3 Full length firm elastic stockings or tights; also special anti–G trousers.

Chorea

Most choreiform movements seen in elderly patients are drug-induced (see Table 11.4). However orofacial dyskinesia is also seen in the absence of an incriminating drug history. Other choreas to be aware of are:

1 Senile chorea

This is rare in a setting of normal intellect. It is more commonly associated with some other disorder such as SDAT or cerebrovascular disease. Some cases may actually be occult Huntington's chorea.

2 Huntington's chorea

An autosomal dominant inherited disease, which sometimes becomes manifest very late in life. There is gradual onset of bilateral symmetrical chorea and dementia.

3 Infarction of the basal ganglia

This may produce a unilateral or asymmetrical chorea of sudden onset. Usually it settles spontaneously but if it fails to do so and is severe, consider stereotactic surgery.

Dystonias other than torticollis are rare in late life.

Primary cerebellar degeneration

A slowly progressive disorder of later life with dysarthria, intention tremor and ataxia, but usually no nystagmus. Other points to note are:

1 It may be of hereditary or sporadic aetiology.
2 Voluntary power is preserved despite the hypotonia.
3 Mental deterioration and loss of sphincter control occurs in advanced cases.
4 The differential diagnosis should include:
• Malignant disease both metastatic and non-metastatic.
• Subacute combined degeneration of the spinal cord.

Restless legs syndrome (Ekbom's syndrome)

This consists of an unpleasant creeping sensation with occasionally, painful cramps and nocturnal myoclonus, as well as aches and pains in leg muscles at rest. The symptoms are worse at night and may be relieved by walking. The aetiology is unknown and treatment empirical but when associated with an underlying disorder such as iron deficiency anaemia, rheumatoid arthritis, uraemia, hypothyroidism or Parkinson's disease, treatment of that may relieve the restless legs. Otherwise the most effective drugs to try are clonazepam, carbamazepine or chlorpromazine at night. Levodopa with decarboxylase inhibitor has recently been advocated. Akathisia due to drugs should be excluded (see Table 11.4).

Chronic subdural haematoma

This relatively uncommon condition is something of an enigma. It consists of an encysted collection of blood between the dura and arachnoid mater which tends to expand. Old people are at especial risk because of the mobility of a shrunken brain within the skull and the frequency of falls. A very high index of suspicion is required to spot these eminently treatable cases in 'run-of-the-mill' geriatric hospital admissions where intracranial tumour is much more common and cerebrovascular disease is infinitely more common. Clinically:

1 Head injury is reported in one-half of cases but may be trivial.
2 Persistent symptoms develop after an interval of days or weeks.
3 Patients present with one or more of the following:
• Ingravescent or completed hemiparesis, often mild.
• Drowsiness, headache or personality change.
• Intellectual impairment with marked fluctuation over hours or days in a minority of cases (about 20 per cent).

Management
1 A plain film of the skull is of limited value but may show fracture or displacement of midline structures, however bilateral haematomata are fairly common. Scintiscan and/or CT are usually diagnostic.
2 In a patient who was previously mentally normal, evacuation of a sizeable expanding haematoma can be expected to give much improvement.
3 Shallow, non-progressive lesions do not show benefit from neurosurgery.
4 Some cases resolve spontaneously.

Intracranial tumours

Intracranial (IC) tumours are much less common than stroke or PD but are found in the elderly more often than in younger adults. Primary tumours may be benign (meningioma) or malignant (glioma). The prevalence is difficult to assess because many are asymptomatic, misdiagnosed or diagnosed only at autopsy which is performed for some other condition.

Metastases account for some 40–50 per cent of intracranial tumours in this age group. They may be multiple, affecting the hemispheres or cerebellum but rarely the brain stem. The primary will be in the lung in two-thirds of cases but other sites include the breast, colon, rectum, kidney and melanoma of the skin or eye. Metastases present a clinical picture similar to glioblastoma multiforme and the prognosis is grim.

Clinical presentations

Hemisphere lesion
1 Progressive, smooth or fluctuating neurological deficit over weeks or months in about 80 per cent of cases and/or
2 Intellectual impairment or personality change which is much more rapid than senile dementia in about 40 per cent cases, or
3 Acute onset hemiplegia in about 5 per cent of cases.
4 May also have epilepsy, drowsiness, headache, rarely papilloedema.

Posterior fossa lesion
1 Ataxia with cerebellar signs.

2 Intellectual impairment, urinary incontinence, long-tract signs.

3 Headache, raised IC pressure, obstructive hydrocephalus.

Raised IC pressure occurs much later in old people and its recognition is bedevilled by the paucity or absence of characteristic symptoms and signs, including papilloedema. The patient simply 'goes off' with apathy, confusion, increasing immobility and incontinence.

Diagnosis of intracranial tumour

1 Plain radiograph of the skull may or may not be helpful.

2 If the clinical picture is suggestive, CT or radionuclide imaging will confirm or refute the diagnosis.

3 Lumbar puncture is hazardous if IC pressure is raised and this may not be evident.

Treatment

1 Surgery is indicated for benign, accessible growths and for the relief of obstructive hydrocephalus.

2 High dose steroid therapy is sometimes valuable for short-term palliation in about 50 per cent of IC malignancies.

Neurological and myopathic complications of malignant disease

Malignancy is an ever-present possibility in the neurology of the aged. Apart from primary tumours of the nervous system, metastases frequently account for malignant intracranial lesions and deposits in the spine, where they cause pathological fractures and cord compression, a neurological emergency. The primary growth may not be apparent but bronchus and breast should always be considered. Additionally, the CNS may be involved from a distant primary even in the absence of metastases. The mechanisms are obscure but presumed to be 'toxic', metabolic or due to an abnormal immune response. The main clinical pictures to consider are:

1 Symmetrical peripheral neuropathy, especially sensory.

2 Subacute cerebellar degeneration which is more rapid than in primary cerebellar degeneration.

3 Myopathy, especially proximal and starting in the thighs.

4 Cerebral atrophy causing dementia which progresses more rapidly than SDAT.

5 A disorder resembling rapid onset of motor neurone disease.

Treatment is that of the primary lesion but even its complete ablation is no guarantee of neurological recovery.

Normal pressure hydrocephalus (NPH)

Normal pressure hydrocephalus is a disorder of later life characterized by enlarged ventricles but with a cerebrospinal fluid (CSF) pressure which is normal or low, i.e. less than 180 mm H_2O. Classically there is a fairly rapid onset of:

1 Dementia.
2 Gait disturbance.
3 Incontinence.

It is possible that the CSF was earlier at higher pressure, falling as the ventricles dilate.

Management

Other remediable causes of dementia should be excluded. CT is the most valuable investigation. The ventricles will be enlarged but with little or no cortical atrophy. A shunting procedure should be considered, but not all cases respond and the complication rate is about 30–40 per cent. The more typical the CT appearances the greater the potential value of the operation.

Herpes zoster

Herpes zoster is a reactivation of a dormant varicella infection affecting the peripheral sensory neurone and the area of skin supplied. Occasionally the anterior horn cells are also involved causing muscle wasting. More than one adjacent segment may be affected. The cumulative incidence is very high so that about half of the population is affected eventually.

Aetiology

1 A childhood varicella infection is reactivated decades later.
2 Susceptibility increases sharply with age as a result of waning immunity (idiopathic zoster) and elderly females are especially at risk.
3 Impaired immunity may be due to diseases such as myeloma and lymphatic leukaemia or to the use of immunosuppressive drugs (symptomatic zoster).

Clinical picture
This includes:
1 Initial general malaise with fever and chills.
2 A prodrome of pain, paraesthesia and hyperaesthesia in the distribution of one or more dorsal roots, most often thoracic (over 50 per cent) or trigeminal (10–15 per cent) lasting a few days.
3 A characteristic vesicular rash in the affected dermatome(s) appears.
4 Involvement of the eye if the ophthalmic division of the trigeminal nerve is affected.
5 Post-herpetic neuralgia in more than half of elderly victims.
6 Rare but very serious complications, which are more likely to occur in the symptomatic cases, e.g. generalized varicella, pneumonia or encephalitis.

Treatment
Treatment advocated in the acute phase includes:
1 Analgesics. Also a short, relatively high-dose course of prednisolone given early may relieve pain in severe cases.
2 Topical application of 40 per cent idoxuridine in dimethylsulphoxide as soon as the rash appears.
3 High-dose acyclovir orally or intravenously, preferably in the prodomal stage and not later than 48 hours after the appearance of the rash. Reduce the dose if there is evidence of impaired renal function.
4 Urgent referral to the ophthalmologist, if there is eye involvement, regarding use of local atropine, idoxuridine, prednisolone and acyclovir.

Persistent post-herpetic neuralgia
Intractable neuralgia is the unsolved problem in the management of herpes zoster. Present guidelines include:
1 Avoid addictive drugs.
2 Antidepressants or phenothiazines are useful and potentiate mild to moderate analgesics.
3 Anticonvulsants are worth trying.
4 Physical therapies, such as cold sprays, electrical vibrators and transcutaneous nerve stimulation, may help in the otherwise intractable case.
5 Referral to pain clinic if severe and persistent.

Motor neurone disease

A degeneration of the anterior horn cells, motor cranial nuclei and the pyramidal tracts with a prevalence range of 2.5–7/100000. Age of onset is usually between 50 and 70 years.

Clinical features
1 A mixed picture is most often found; especially upper motor neurone signs in legs and lower motor neurone signs in arms and a mixture of the two in the bulbar muscles.
2 Absence of evidence of peripheral neuropathy, e.g. sensory loss.

Treatment
Nil specific but compassionate supportive measures, psychological as well as physical, are required for patient and carers.

Peripheral polyneuropathy

Peripheral polyneuropathy has a very high incidence in late life, approaching 90 per cent in elderly diabetics (see Fig. 11.1).

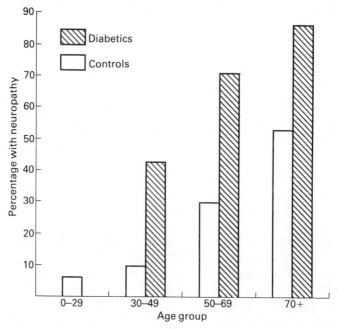

Fig. 11.1. Peripheral neuropathy.

Although nerve conduction velocity falls with age clinical neuropathy must be regarded as due to disease even if the cause is not evident. The clinical signs are usually much less dramatic than the symptoms of pain, loss of sensation, ataxia and ANS dysfunction.

Aetiology
Most cases remain 'idiopathic' or undiagnosed, but consider especially:

1 Metabolic—diabetes mellitus (the most common cause), alcohol, renal failure, amyloid and dysproteinaemia.

2 Carcinoma—especially bronchial, the neoplasm may be occult.

3 Drugs, e.g. nitrofurantoin, metronidazole, isoniazid, vincristine.

4 Vitamin B complex deficiencies, e.g. from inadequate diet or pernicious anaemia.

5 Other causes—the Guillain–Barré syndrome and connective tissue disease.

Trigeminal neuralgia (tic douloureux)

This distressing disorder is rare before the age of 50. It especially affects women and is characterized by brief but recurrent paroxysms of pain in one or more divisions of the fifth cranial nerve. Carbamazepine is the drug of first choice but neurosurgical referral may be required.

Drop attacks

These attacks occur in 3–4 per cent of elderly women. The victim drops to the ground without warning and with no loss of consciousness and no neurological deficit has been recorded. Once on the ground most can get up unaided almost immediately but others are unable to rise to their feet although there is no paralysis. If stood up, although much shaken by the experience, usually she can walk with little or no help. Pressure on the soles of the feet possibly reactivates the failed antigravity reflexes. The aetiology is obscure but transient vertebrobasilar ischaemia leading to loss of postural reflexes has been postulated. No effective method of prevention other than that for the avoidance of orthostatic hypotension (Chapter 12) can be suggested.

Autonomic nervous system (ANS) dysfunction

The reactivity of the autonomic nervous system (ANS) is generally less efficient in both onset and recovery time in elderly people. Control over homeostatic mechanisms is weakened (see Chapter 15) and sinus arrhythmia is often considerably reduced or absent. Gross ANS dysfunction occurs from disease or drug treatment affecting receptors, transmission in peripheral nerves, autonomic ganglia and central CNS connections, and effector organs. Common impairments of control in old age relate to:

1 Body temperature.
2 Systemic blood pressure.
3 Gastrointestinal motility.
4 Bladder motility.

The most common cause of ANS dysfunction is diabetes mellitus but a variety of other possibilities must be kept in mind (see Table 11.5). Clinical features of ANS dysfunction include:

• Orthostatic hypotension (see Chapter 12).
• Dysphagia, delayed gastric emptying, diarrhoea, constipation.

Table 11.5. Pathological conditions affecting autonomic function

Central	Peripheral
Cerebrovascular disease	Diabetes mellitus
Parkinsonism	Malignancy, especially bronchus and pancreas
Shy–Drager syndrome	Amyloidosis
Chronic alcoholism	Chronic alcoholism
Psychotropic drugs, especially phenothiazines	Peripheral acting drugs, e.g. beta-blockers
Paraplegia	Acute infective polyneuropathy
Wernicke's encephalopathy	Vitamin B complex deficiency, including pernicious anaemia
Tabes dorsalis	

(Adapted from Exton–Smith 1982)

- Liability to hypothermia (see Chapter 15).
- Atonic bladder leading to retention of urine.
- Disorders of pupillary reflexes, especially failure to dilate in the dark.
- Abnormalities of vasomotor reflexes and of sweating (anhidrosis, hyperhidrosis).
- Impotence.

Management

1 Remove or control the cause where possible, e.g. alcohol, drugs, vitamin B complex deficiency.
2 Apply appropriate measures to combat the liability to hypothermia, orthostatic hypotension, bladder and bowel disturbances, as outlined elsewhere in this book.
3 Assess severity of ANS dysfunction.

Tests of autonomic function

These simple tests are based on assessment of cardiovascular reflexes, are non-invasive and do not require highly specialized equipment. To be valid there should be no cardiac failure or arrhythmia. They cannot localize the site of the ANS defect but test the whole reflex including receptor and end-organ responses.

Parasympathetic

HEART RATE VARIATION (HRV) DURING DEEP BREATHING
Performed most easily using an instantaneous cardiac rate meter but can use ECG and measure R–R intervals. The difference between maximum and minimum heart rates before and after six deep breaths in the lying or sitting position is the HRV. Normally greater than 15 beats per minute in healthy young people it tends to fall with age and below 10 is regarded as abnormal. Absence of sinus arrhythmia on ECG has a similar significance.

HEART RATE RESPONSE TO STANDING
The subject stands up, or is put upright on a tilting table, after 2 minutes rest in the lying position, and the change in heart rate is measured by continuous ECG. The maximal rate is usually around the 15th beat and minimal around the 30th. The lengths of the R–R intervals at these points are measured with a ruler from the ECG and the 30 to 15 ratio calculated. Normally the ratio is 1.03 or greater but

declines somewhat with age. Values of 1.0 and less are abnormal. Tests 1 and 2 principally depend upon the integrity of the vagus.

Sympathetic

BLOOD PRESSURE RESPONSE TO STANDING
This test can be combined conveniently with the two above. Normally the systolic BP falls no more than 15 mm Hg, the diastolic falls or rises a little and the mean arterial blood pressure is virtually unchanged. The main homeostatic mechanism is said to be sympathetic splanchnic vasoconstriction. In many elderly people the state of the vasculature (including the presence of varicose veins) and the prescribed medication are of more importance in causing a pressure drop than ANS dysfunction. There is no general agreement regarding an abnormal fall in pressure but if symptoms occur, the same management as that regarding orthostatic hypotension may be beneficial (see Chapter 12).

Other tests
The heart rate response to the Valsalva manoeuvre (parasympathetic) and the BP response to sustained handgrip (sympathetic) are not generally useful in geriatric practice because of difficulties in patient cooperation. In suitably equipped centres thermoregulatory function and the BP response to lower-body negative pressure can be tested with minimal patient cooperation.

Further reading

Caird F.I. (ed.) (1982) *Neurological Disorders in the Elderly*. Wright, Bristol.
Collins K.J. (1983) Automatic failure and the elderly. In: Bannister R. *Autonomic Failure*, pp. 488–507. OUP, Oxford.
Exton-Smith A.N. (1982) Disorders of the autonomic system. In: Caird F.I. (ed.) *Neurological Disorders in the Elderly*. Wright, Bristol.
Godfrey J.B. & Caird F.I. (1984) Intracranial tumours in the elderly. *Age and Ageing*, **13**, 152–8.
Oxtoby M. (1982) Parkinson's disease patients and their social needs. Parkinson's Disease Society, London.

Useful addresses

Alzheimer Disease Society, 3rd Floor, Bank Building, Fulham Broadway, London SW6 1EP.
Parkinson's Disease Society, 36 Portland Place, London W1N 3DG.

Chapter 12
Cardiovascular Disease

Age changes

1 Structure
(a) Lipofuscin accumulates in myocardial cells and amyloid deposits are found extracellularly.
(b) There is a loss and fragmentation of vessel wall elastin leading to diminished distensibility.
(c) Calcification commences in aortic valve cusps and the mitral valve ring.
(d) The length and breadth of the aorta continues to increase throughout life.

2 Function
(a) Cardiac output declines.
(b) Maximum heart rate declines.
(c) Stroke volume declines.
(d) The arteriovenous oxygen gradient rises.
(e) Resting and maximal oxygen consumption falls linearly with age. The latter is one of the best measures of the functional state and the decline is 1 per cent per annum, and for the average 70–75-year-old female simply walking at 5 km/hour represents maximal aerobic exercise. Regular exercise can reverse this decline by 10 years.
(f) The myocardial response to beta stimulation decreases.

Common findings

The apex beat
A laterally displaced apex beat is a commonplace physical sign in geriatric medicine and a cardiothoracic ratio greater than 50 per cent is found on chest X-rays of 70 per cent of women over 70. This probably overestimates a change in heart size since the chest may

distort in many old people. Kyphoscoliosis renders location of the apex an unreliable indication of heart size.

Atrial fibrillation

Atrial fibrillation, like most other abnormal findings, is much commoner in elderly hospital patients (22 per cent) than in population surveys in which it is the established heart rhythm in 5–11 per cent of people aged 75 and over, but about a third of nonagenarians. It is a very important abnormality because non-rheumatic atrial fibrillation (NRAF) in an apparently healthy heart seems to be associated with a 4- to 5-fold increase in the risk of stroke and between the ages of 80 and 89, 36 per cent of all strokes occur in patients with fibrillation. One survey found this rhythm in 40 per cent of women over 65 admitted with stroke. It remains unclear whether this is generally due to embolization from intra-atrial thrombus formation, whether the fibrillation is merely a marker of widespread arterial disease, or whether indeed fibrillation with its varying rate leads to periods of low cerebral perfusion when vulnerable territory supplied by diseased vessels is liable to infarction. The mortality following a stroke is also higher, and there is also a high incidence of atrial fibrillation in patients with multi-infarct dementia. A considerable proportion of aged fibrillators do not require digoxin because concomitant conduction system disease prevents the ventricular rate becoming excessively rapid. In only a small minority of cases is atrial fibrillation due to thyrotoxicosis.

The 24-hour ambulatory rhythm tape

Transient disturbances of heart rate and rhythm may cause disturbances of cerebral function sometimes resulting in falls or syncopal attacks. Unfortunately, the incidence of these episodes increases with age and false positives are thus likely unless carefully correlated with symptoms on the diary card or event button. In the absence of such correlation, bursts of abnormal rhythm may at best be regarded as markers. The occurrence of numerous ectopic beats is seldom of any significance although salvoes may point towards runs of tachyarrhythmia. The symptoms are seldom of daily occurrence so false negatives are also common. If in doubt concerning the significance of short runs of tachycardia, the best way forward is a therapeutic trial of anti-arrhythmic treatment.

The systolic murmur

Surveys report that 30–60 per cent of elderly patients have systolic murmurs arising from abnormal heart valves and the proportion rises at more advanced ages. It is not always easy to be sure on clinical grounds, but the murmur originates from the mitral valve in about 50 per cent of cases, the aortic valve in 25 per cent and both are abnormal in another 25 per cent.

Mitral regurgitation

This condition is thought to be associated with some cases of transient cerebral or retinal ischaemia. The commonest causes in elderly people are:

Calcification of mitral ring
Dilatation of left ventricle and mitral ring
Mucoid (myxomatous) degeneration of cusps
Floppy mitral valve with prolapse of posterior cusp
Papillary muscle dysfunction—usually ischaemic
Rupture of chordae tendinae (often partial)
Infective endocarditis
Rheumatic heart disease

Calcific aortic stenosis

This is the most important disease of the aged aortic valve, and may cause angina, breathlessness and syncope or pre-syncopal attacks. These features should make the physician consider seeking echo-cardiography with a view to valve replacement or, more recently, balloon dilatation in frailer subjects. Mixed aortic valve disease is frequently encountered.

Common conditions

Complete heart block—indications for pacemaker:
1 Stokes–Adams attacks are an indication for urgent pacing.
2 Persistent failure, lethargy, or poor exercise tolerance are indications for pacing.
3 In the absence of these indications, practice varies widely, and some would argue that all cases of chronic third degree block should be paced while others would select patients with a ventricular rate below 40.

4 Impaired cerebration, unless clearly coinciding with the onset of heart block, rarely responds to pacing. A trial of longacting isoprenaline (Saventrine) to speed up the ventricular rate or a temporary pacing wire may help to determine the likely response.

Physicians are sometimes puzzled when a patient with a normally functioning ventricular pacemaker develops symptoms such as syncope, dizziness, breathlessness, chest pain, fatigue and palpitations. This may be due to the pacemaker syndrome in which retrograde a–v conduction causes atrial contractions against closed a–v valves with a rise in pressure and a drop in cardiac output and blood pressure: cannon waves may be seen. This does not occur in dual chamber pacing. The patient should be referred back to the cardiologist.

Heart failure
Both congestive cardiac failure (CCF) and left ventricular failure (LVF) are common in the elderly. CCF is thought to affect 5 per cent of people over 65, and the causes are given below. It should be emphasized that oedema of the ankles is often non-cardiac in origin (chairbound immobility, drug-induced fluid retention). Acute breathlessness may simply be due to LVF but an infective element is often present and superimposed airway obstruction is a common complication. An important differential diagnosis is pulmonary embolic disease. Treatment of sinus rhythm heart failure is with diuretics. If angiotensin-converting enzyme (ACE) inhibitors are necessary, the dose of diuretics should be reviewed. Causes of congestive cardiac failure:

Ischaemic heart disease
Hypertension
Valvular heart disease
Cor pulmonale including pulmonary thromboembolism
Thyrotoxicosis
Severe anaemia
Arrhythmia due to conduction tissue fibrosis
Drugs
Cardiomyopathy

Angina
Angina is common in the elderly and requires little comment except to state that there are numerous reports, especially from the USA,

of coronary artery bypass graft surgery being performed on patients in their late seventies with unstable angina when medical measures have failed. A mortality of 4 or 5 per cent has been quoted and although there are more non-fatal perioperative complications and a slightly longer hospital stay than in younger age groups, the results have been excellent.

Myocardial infarction

Presentation in the aged is often atypical but by no means always so, and some presenting clinical pictures are as follows:

'Typical' chest pain (20 per cent)
Sudden death
Mild chest discomfort, sometimes attributed to indigestion
'Silent' (previous unidentified episode picked up on ECG)
Heart failure, shortness of breath
Arrhythmia
'Going off', 'failure to thrive'
A fall, found lying on floor, hypotension
Stroke
Confusion
Peripheral gangrene

Cardiopulmonary resuscitation (CPR)

It has generally been found that age alone is a much poorer determinant of outcome than the nature of the abnormal rhythm and the length of the delay before the initiation of effective CPR. Its use selectively but positively will benefit some patients.

It need hardly be said that CPR is only appropriate in the event of abrupt arrest and not simply because death has occurred. A recent survey found a surprising degree of awareness and acceptance of CPR among older subjects. Because the condition of elderly patients changes quickly, it is not usually practical to state in the case notes wether a given patient is a candidate for CPR or not, and if the attending nurse or doctor is in doubt, the decision must be 'go'.

Blood pressure (BP: systolic, diastolic and mean = SBP, DBP, MBP)

Measurement
Indirect methods of measurement are probably reasonably reliable in elderly people despite suggestions to the contrary. The BP may

be more labile in older people, repeated measurements are desirable to obtain true levels, and there is much to be said for taking readings with the patients standing or at least sitting upright.

Levels in elderly subjects
Confusion between normal age changes and an increased incidence of disease reigns supreme. The following tentative statements reflect the current state of the art:

1 In developed countries, cross-sectional studies show the SBP rising until the 70s and then levelling off or fractionally declining, and the DBP rising more gently and levelling off earlier in the 60s so the pulse pressure widens (Figs. 12.1, 12.2 and 12.3). It is uncertain how much of this levelling is due to accelerated attrition among hypertensives. This rise, which is due to an increase in the peripheral resistance, is not inevitable since it appears not to occur in Fijians or in Amazonian Amerindians.

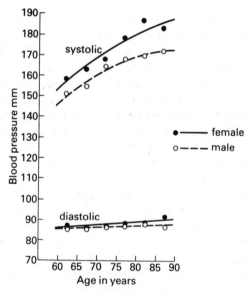

Fig. 12.1. The means of systolic and diastolic blood pressures for females and males for each five-year age group of the sample together with the fitted curves (Source: Anderson W. F. & Cowan N. R. [1959] Arterial pressure in healthy older people. *Clinical Science*, **18**, 103).

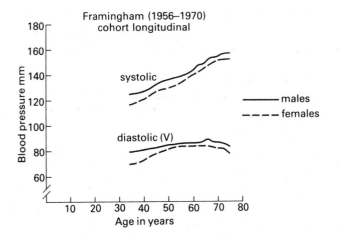

Fig. 12.2. Relationship between age and median population blood pressure levels by sex (Source: Whelton P. K., Hypertension in the elderly. In: Andres R., Bierman E. & Hazzard W. [eds] *Principles of Geriatric Medicine*. McGraw–Hill Book Co., New York).

2 An American survey found the average BP over the age of 65 to be 149/83. At 72, the European Working Party on Hypertension in the Elderly (EWPHE) found an average level of 183/101. In Western societies, the prevalence of hypertension (over 160/95) in the age group 75–79 has been found to be as high as 41–42 per cent. Isolated systolic hypertension (ISH: SBP over 160, DBP 95 or below) affects 25–30 per cent of people over 70. Diastolic hypertension, however, is only present in about 13 per cent of people over 70 or less if repeated readings are taken.

3 Surveys of hypertension as a risk factor have yielded conflicting results, the trend being to confirm an association between a raised SBP and increased cardiovascular mortality and morbidity up to age 74 but not necessarily beyond, and possibly an inverse relationship over age 85. In general, the Framingham study has been much more positive in this regard than have surveys from the UK which have often recruited older populations. Subjects with multi-infarct dementia have been shown to have higher BPs than those with SDAT.

Results of treatment

Of the recent major trials, only EWPHE contained significant

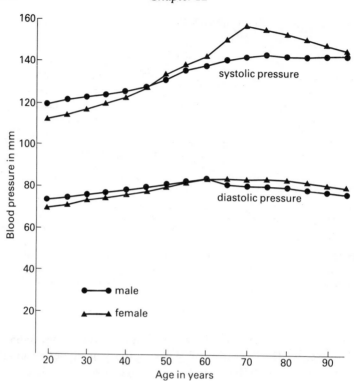

Fig. 12.3. Blood pressure changes in apparently healthy men and women with advancing age. (Source: Maclennan W. J. [1986] The epidemiology of hypertension in the elderly. In: Tallis R. C. & Caird F. I. [eds] *Advanced Geriatric Medicine*, **5** Churchill Livingstone, Edinburgh. Fig. 10.1, p. 80, adapted from Hickler R. B. [1983] Aging and hypertension. In: *Journal of the American Geriatric Society*, **31**, 421).

numbers of men and women well into their 70s. A repeated SBP of 160 or over and DBP of 90 or over qualified for entry: ISH did not and the results do not apply to it. Cardiovascular events, fatal plus non-fatal, were reduced by 36 per cent in the treated group, cardio-vascular deaths by 27 per cent and total mortality by 26 per cent. Ninety patients had to be treated for 1 year to avoid 1 stroke (although it should be noted that cardiac deaths were reduced by 47 per cent). Numbers of patients of 80 or over were probably too few to base treatment strategies on, and many would hesitate to draw definite conclusions about the benefits to patients over 75.

Who should be treated?
Accelerated hypertension clearly requires treatment but is most uncommon in this age group. End-organ damage might be regarded as an indication for treatment, but is difficult to identify since LVH, retinal arterial changes and impaired renal function are so common and non-specific. 'Graduate' hypertensives who are well on their long-term treatment are taken off it at the doctor's peril. Otherwise, we would restrict therapy to those under 75 with substantiated hypertension and would start with a diuretic and use a calcium antagonist as the second line of treatment. It is important to remember that 'hypertension is an asymptomatic disease in the elderly, and should remain so when treated'. Also, the final confession of ignorance: hypertension can only be defined as 'the level of blood pressure at which the patient's health would benefit from treatment'.

Orthostatic (postural) hypotension

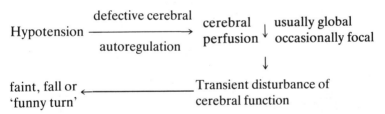

Hypotension is poorly tolerated by the old and can have serious consequences. If the usual definition of orthostatic hypotension as a fall of over 20 mm in the SBP or 10 mm in the DBP is accepted, then a prevalence of 20–30 per cent in community-living elderly people has been recorded. There may be a convincing history correlating the often rather vague symptoms with getting out of bed in the night or on waking, but a modest drop in BP, such as that given above, may clearly be an incidental finding. It is much more likely to be of clinical significance if the manoeuvre is accompanied by distress.
Causes of orthostatic hypotension include the following:
    Hypovolaemia due to salt and water depletion
    Autonomic nervous system dysfunction (Chapter 11)

Drugs—antihypertensives including diuretics
        phenothiazines
        antidepressants
        levodopa
        vasodilators (including alcohol)
        narcotic analgesics
        verapamil
        disopyramide
Prolonged recumbency
Cardiac disease (e.g. infarction)

The treatment of orthostatic hypotension is as follows:

Correct cause if identified

Advise concerning sensible precautions ('have a bath with a friend')

Compression hosiery—full length, preferably tights

Medication—fludrocortisone, pindolol, indomethacin and dihydroergotamine have been tried

Head up tilt to bed (20°) to reduce nocturnal diuresis.

Postprandial hypotension

Similar falls in SBP have been noted in some elderly subjects 30–60 minutes after eating a meal. Sometimes they are associated with syncopal or presyncopal attacks. Exertional hypotension is another occasional finding and there is some evidence that certain subjects are liable to apparently random transient falls in blood pressure without obvious circulatory causes such as arrhythmia, minor gastrointestinal bleeds or small pulmonary emboli. Hypotension is sometimes a component additional to bradycardia and/or heart block in the syncope of carotid sinus hypersensitivity.

Infective endocarditis

The mortality remains 15–30 per cent, the annual number of deaths in England and Wales is about 200, and the majority are now patients aged 60 or more. Previously unrecognized calcific valve disease is the major risk factor in Western countries. *Strep. viridans* is the commonest organism, and dental and genito-urinary procedures should be covered with prophylactic antibiotics although it is not clear which other invasive activities should be covered. Patients with prosthetic heart valves require scrupulous prophylaxis for even trivial procedures.

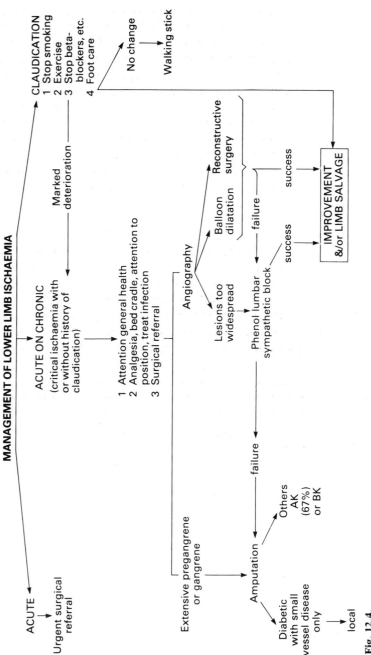

MANAGEMENT OF LOWER LIMB ISCHAEMIA

ACUTE → Urgent surgical referral

ACUTE ON CHRONIC (critical ischaemia with or without history of claudication)

1 Attention general health
2 Analgesia, bed cradle, attention to position, treat infection
3 Surgical referral

CLAUDICATION
1 Stop smoking
2 Exercise
3 Stop beta-blockers, etc.
4 Foot care

Marked deterioration

No change → Walking stick

Angiography

Reconstructive surgery
Balloon dilatation
Lesions too widespread → Phenol lumbar sympathetic block

failure

success → IMPROVEMENT &/or LIMB SALVAGE
success

Extensive pregangrene or gangrene → Amputation

Others AK (67%) or BK

Diabetic with small vessel disease only → local

Fig. 12.4.

Abdominal aortic aneurysm

By definition, the aneurysmal aorta is over 3.5 cm in diameter and wider than at any proximal point. It is when a diameter of 6 cm is reached (as imaged by ultrasound) that the risk of rupture rapidly increases and elective surgery is advised in otherwise suitable subjects simply because the surgical risk, when the patient is admitted as an emergency, is horrendous. A 7 cm aneurysm has a 20 per cent risk of rupture within 12 months and over 60 per cent within 5 years. The elective operative mortality is 2–10 per cent.

Peripheral vascular disease

Claudication is common but it is important to be alert to the fact that the housebound and immobile will not give a history of claudication even in the presence of severe lower limb ischaemia. Under these circumstances, the first manifestation of the disease is likely to be critical ischaemia (rest pain, ulcers, or necrotic or septic skin lesions), perhaps following chiropody or trauma or a fall in perfusion due to cardiac or pulmonary disease. If pre-gangrenous changes develop rapidly, an embolus may be suspected and fruitlessly sought because the haemodynamic crisis in the presence of occlusive arterial disease has resulted in a marginally perfused foot becoming unviable. In all patients in whom the foot pulses are impalpable, therefore, Doppler measurements of ankle systolic pressure will provide a very useful base line and the presence of pulses higher up the limb and of bruits anywhere from the aorta to the popliteal artery should be recorded. Scrupulous care should be taken of the poorly perfused foot. The management of lower limb ischaemia is outlined in Fig. 12.4. If amputation is required, the objectives are, (1) to save life, (2) to relieve pain, and (3) to make rehabilitation possible. It should therefore be seen as a positive form of treatment and is mandatory in all patients with gangrene unless imminently terminal.

Giant cell arteritis

The features of this disease are given below. The response to high dose corticosteroids is dramatic. After a year or 18 months, it may be possible to withdraw them with extreme circumspection in patients under 70 or 75, monitoring symptoms and the ESR.

Patients in their eighties may be better left on a small dose for life. Features include:

Late age of onset

Pathology—thickening of intima, giant cell infiltration

Polymyalgia rheumatica (Chapter 9)

Headache

Scalp tenderness

Tender, thickened superficial temporal arteries

Constitutional—fever, weight loss, anaemia, high ESR

Occlusion of short posterior ciliary artery with blindness

Jaw claudication

Pain in tongue

Stroke

Coronary artery involvement

Peripheral arterial involvement

'Going off', 'failure to thrive'

Anaemia, abnormal liver function tests

Venous thromboembolic disease

Thirty per cent of aged general surgical patients, 60 per cent of stroke victims and 75 per cent of old ladies with femoral neck fracture will develop a deep vein thrombosis (DVT) unless prophylactic measures are taken. Of those confined to below the knee, 25 per cent will later extend above the knee, of which half will embolize. DVT should be confirmed by venography if in doubt and even if localized to the calf should therefore be treated with warfarin for 3 months unless there are contraindications. Pulmonary embolism warrants anticoagulation for at least this period and perhaps 6 months since the mortality is about a third without treatment but under 10 per cent with it. It is a geriatric master of disguise (see below) and if the possibility is considered an isotope V/Q scan can be enormously helpful.

Pulmonary embolism—presentation:

Typical—pleuritic pain, haemoptysis

Collapse

Sudden death

Fever

Breathless attacks

Arrhythmia

Cough, 'pneumonia'

Bronchospasm
Pulmonary oedema
Increasing exertional dyspnoea
'Going off', failure to thrive', hypotension
Confusion
Falls

Further reading

Anon (1985) Presentation of myocardial infarction in the elderly. *Lancet*, **ii**, 1077–8.

Anon (1986) Is lone atrial fibrillation really benign? *Lancet*, **i**, 305–6.

Dall J.L.C. (1981) Ischaemic heart disease in the elderly. In: Reinders–Folmer A.M.J. & Schouten J. (eds) *Geriatrics for the Practitioner, Excerpta Medica*, pp.53–60, Amsterdam.

Klauser S.C. & Schwartz A.B. (1985) The aging heart. *Clinics in Geriatric Medicine*, **1**, 119–42.

Luchi R.J. & Ware T. (1985) Congestive heart failure. In: Isaacs B. (ed.) *Recent Advances in Geriatric Medicine*, **3**, pp. 19–36. Churchill Livingstone, Edinburgh.

MacLennan W.J., Swales J.D., Williams B.O. & Orme M.l'E. (1986) Hypertension in the elderly. In: Tallis R.C. & Caird F.I. (eds) *Advanced Geriatric Medicine*, **5**, pp. 79–106. Churchill Livingstone, Edinburgh.

Mulley G.P. (1982) Giant cell arteritis. *British Journal of Hospital Medicine*, **27**, 413–6.

Watson R.D.S. (1987) Treating postural hypotension. *British Medical Journal*, **294**, 390–1.

Chapter 13
Respiratory Disease

Age changes

1 There is a reduction in lung elasticity and chest wall compliance so that air-trapping leads to a rise in residual volume and a fall in the vital capacity (see Tables 13.1 & 13.2).

Table 13.1. Respiratory function in the elderly—mean values

Age	Sex	FEV 1	FVC
62–70	M	2.18	3.17
	F	1.63	2.02
70–79	M	1.92	2.85
	F	1.43	1.80
80+	M	1.97	2.89
	F	1.01	1.45

(After Milne J.S. & Williamson J. [1972], Respiratory function tests in older people. *Clinical Science* **42**, 371–81. Note—in the original, values are given for different heights. FEV1 = forced expiratory volume in 1 second; FVC = forced vital capacity.)

2 Arterial oxygen tension (PaO_2) falls from 95 mm (12.7 KPa) at age 30 to 75 mm (10 KPa) at 60.
3 Maximum breathing capacity per minute is diminished.
4 Mucociliary protection of the lower airway is impaired.

Influenza

This illness can be very prostrating, especially in old people. Simple tasks such as preparing drinks and washing, may be too much effort and general weakness may lead to a fall. Those with chronic disease,

141

Table 13.2. Peak expiratory flow rate (l/min) in elderly subjects: predicted values

Height	1.50m 4'11''	1.55m 5'1''	1.6m 5'3	1.65m 5'5''	1.7m 5'7''	1.75m 5'9''	1.80m 5'11''
Age							
65	443	468	483	498	513	528	543
	311	330	349	367	386	405	424
70	435	449	464	478	493	507	522
	301	320	338	357	376	394	413
75	423	438	452	466	480	494	508
	290	309	328	346	365	384	403
80	412	426	440	453	467	481	495
	280	299	317	336	355	373	392
85	410	414	428	441	454	468	481
	269	288	307	325	344	363	382

Upper figures are for males and lower for females. (After Cotes J.E. *Lung Function*, [1979] 4th ed. Blackwell Scientific Publications, Oxford)

especially chronic bronchitis, diabetes, heart failure or renal failure are more prone to develop pneumonia, and this may be due to *H. influenzae* or *Strep. pneumoniae* but is quite likely to be staphyloccal.

Very frail, aged persons resident in institutions form another group highly susceptible to outbreaks of 'flu, which sometimes lead to a high mortality, although principally among those whose hold on life is exceedingly precarious and who have owed months or even years of extra life to the institutions which cared for them.

'Flu vaccine should be offered to all those who come into the two categories referred to above, unless there is a history of allergy. Immunity takes 2–4 weeks to develop and lasts 6–8 months, so vaccination is carried out in September or October every year. It affords protection to 60–90 per cent of those immunized. Occasionally a supplementary vaccine against a specific currently prevalent strain has to be prepared later in the year, and should be offered to the same high risk groups of patients.

Pneumonia

This forms a large part of the caseload in general and hospital practice, and the diagnosis is often difficult with tachypnoea being a valuable clinical pointer. A respiratory rate of over 30 is an ominous sign. Acute confusion is another common feature and is also associated with a poor prognosis. A number of patients present with a fall as the initial feature of their illness, and tachycardia and hypotension are frequent findings. Some common forms of pneumonia with their therapeutic implications are given in Table 13.3. Older people often swallow their sputum, and blood cultures may offer the only opportunity of identifying the organism.

Table 13.3. Common types of pneumonia in the old

1 'Clean, off the street'	Probably pneumococcal but possibilities include haemophilus, staphylococcus, legionella, mycoplasma: hence use erythromycin (initially IV if patient very unwell)
2 Complicating chronic obstructive airways disease	High risk of respiratory failure—requires O_2 by venturi mask, nebulized beta-2 adrenergic bronchodilator, possibly steroids, in addition to amoxycillin or Augmentin
3 Complicating influenza	Suspect staphylococcus during outbreak of influenza and give flucloxacillin in addition to broad-spectrum antibiotic
4 Aspiration pneumonia	Very common due to prevalence of disorders of deglutition and oesophageal motility and gastro-oesophageal reflux. Use Augmentin and possibly metronidazole in addition
5 Complicating other disorders	It is frequently impossible to be certain if breathlessness is mainly of cardiac or pulmonary origin—if in doubt, treat the patient for both—not forgetting the possibility of pulmonary embolism

Pulmonary tuberculosis

In the Western world, tuberculosis has shifted its offensive towards the older age groups, and in Arkansas in 1981, 51 per cent of cases were 65 or older. Recently it was shown that only 26 per cent of elderly residents of two American chronic disease hospitals had positive tuberculin tests. Thirty per cent of the remainder showed other evidence of anergy and these patients had a higher 1-year mortality rate than positive responders. A recent survey of nursing homes in the US showed that only 10–15 per cent of new entrants were tuberculin positive, but that the proportion had risen to 25 per cent a few months later. This cohort, in the 1930s, had a 70 per cent tuberculin positive rate, suggesting that these aged patients had outlived their tubercle bacilli and had become susceptible to a second primary infection. Reactivation probably remains the commonest cause of active disease, particularly when the host defence is lowered by malnutrition, corticosteroids or concomitant illness. Treatment is with isoniazid and rifampicin for 9 months together with ethambutol for the first two. The patient is usually regarded as infectious only if the sputum is positive to direct smear.

Airway obstruction

This occurs in two main conditions—as a complication of chronic obstructive airways disease (COAD), cigarette-induced, particularly during infective exacerbations, and as late-onset asthma (Table 13.4). The former shows variability from week to week, the latter from hour to hour and a single normal spirometric test confirms a diagnosis of asthma. Late-onset asthma may show a fair response to beta–2 adrenergic bronchodilators although this is less

Table 13.4. Differential diagnosis of wheezing

Feature	COAD	Late-onset asthma
Symptoms present for 4 years or more	virtually all patients	minority
Breathlessness	never goes completely, in most cases	may clear totally
Variability	weekly	hourly—some days clear
Permanent cough and spit (with purulent exacerbations)	+	–
Cigarettes	+(even if not now)	±
Childhood asthma	occasional	often
Precipitated by exercise, hyperventilation	not typical	+
Nocturnal exacerbations	not typical (but may occur in cold bedroom)	typical
Response bronchodilators	–	±
Response steroids	poor to moderate	excellent

dramatic than in younger patients and they frequently cause a marked tachycardia and tremor. In addition, inhalation therapy requires too much coordination for many frail and aged subjects unless the device is automatically actuated by inhalation or is attached to a large chamber (e.g. the Nebuhaler) which makes precise timing unnecessary. In severe attacks, nebulized broncho-dilator therapy and corticosteroids are the sheet-anchors of treatment.

A third group of wheezy patients comprises the lifelong asth-matics who have grown old, and who are generally expert at their own management. The late-onset asthmatic, however, is often a childhood asthmatic who has relapsed in late life; some of these patients develop permanent wheezy dyspnoea even though they have never smoked.

Snoring

Much publicity has recently been accorded to this phenomenon by both medical and national press. It is said to increase in incidence with age and to be associated with a number of problems (see below). So far, it has attracted little attention by geriatricians, either because they are not alert to it or because people who snore do not survive long enough!

Problems associated with snoring:
   Sleep apnoea
   Nocturnal death
   Polycythaemia
   Hypertension
   Pulmonary hypertension
   Cardiac failure
   Arrhythmias
   Somnolence
   Angina
   Mental changes
   Insomnia
   Cerebral infarction
   Marital (or extramarital) disharmony

Possible causative factors:
   COAD

Alcohol
Tobacco
Obesity

Carcinoma of the bronchus

This, the commonest cancer in the UK, is rapidly increasing in frequency in females, and has become mainly a disease of older people (75 per cent over 60 in one series, 66 per cent over 65 in another). The histological classification is into squamous, small or oat cell, adenocarcinoma and anaplastic large-cell types. Surgery offers the possibility of a cure in the squamous variety—IF the patient is fit enough, lung function is good (FEV 1 [see Table 13.1] of 1½ litres or more) and there is no distant spread. Lobectomy at the age of 70 has a mortality of about 15 per cent, and pneumonectomy 30 per cent, and the former procedure is not appropriate for patients over 75 or the latter for patients over 70.

Palliative radiotherapy is effective for superior mediastinal obstruction, chest pain and painful bony metastases, but there is little evidence that radiotherapy can prolong life and it produces very few long-term cures. Chemotherapy sometimes prolongs life.

Chest trauma

The injury which requires special mention in relation to older people is rib fracture which is common after fairly mild trauma or even a coughing fit. The diagnosis relies on the clinical sign of marked local tenderness, rather than on X-rays. In an elderly chronic bronchitic the effect on respiratory function can be profound. Shallow breathing combines with a reluctance to cough to produce sputum retention and lobar or segmental collapse. For this reason effective pain relief with non-narcotic agents is very valuable, and intercostal block with marcain or paravertebral block may offer the best means of achieving this. Fracture of a rib or ribs may lead to more serious complications, such as pneumothorax or haemothorax.

Pleural effusions

Effusions in old age are commonly due to heart failure, pneumonia, pulmonary embolism or malignancy, and other causes come into the 'small print' category. If the cause is self-evidently one of the first three, then treatment is clearcut. If it is a mystery, it is the work of a moment to obtain a specimen of the fluid through an ordinary venepuncture needle to ensure that an empyema is not there, and to send the fluid off for malignant cells and culture including tubercle bacilli. A biopsy, however, is more likely to give a pathological diagnosis. If the effusion is massive and causes a great deal of breathlessness (usually a 'white-out' on the X-ray) a therapeutic aspiration will be required. The cause will almost certainly be a carcinoma and if the fluid keeps re-accumulating, intracavitary tetracycline should be considered after aspiration to dryness.

Further reading

Anon (1985) Snoring and sleepiness. *Lancet,* **ii,** 925–6.
Coni N.K., Davison W. & Reiss B.R. (1986) Chapters 16 The Respiratory system & 17 Infections. In: *The Geriatric Prescriber.* Blackwell Scientific Publications, Oxford.
Stark J.E. & Page R.L. (1981) Respiratory diseases. In: Andrews J. & von Hahn H.P. (eds) *Geriatrics for Everyday Practice,* pp. 15–29. Karger, Basel.

Chapter 14
Gastrointestinal Disease

Gastrointestinal symptoms are common throughout life—and the elderly are certainly not excluded. Structural changes, e.g. hiatus hernia, diverticular disease and gallstones all increase with increasing age. Functional changes also increase, e.g. motility problems in the oesophagus and large bowel and falling acid secretion in the stomach. Almost one-fifth of patients presenting at a geriatric outpatient clinic will have gastrointestinal problems.

Age changes

1 Impairment of sense of smell and taste.
2 Loss of teeth.
3 Impaired coordination of swallowing and oesophageal peristalsis.
4 Reduced gastric acid secretion.
5 Reduced pancreatic function due to duct and parenchymatous changes.
6 Increased development of diverticula.
7 Reduced surface area in small bowel.
8 Reduced large-bowel motility.

Weight loss

1 Ageing changes
There would appear to be a natural tendency to weight loss with increasing age—due to a reduction in body-water content, bone loss (osteoporosis), thinning of connective tissue and the conversion of muscle to fat. However, those who maintain their lean body mass as they advance into old age have a better life expectancy than their shrinking peers.

2 Systemic disease

Weight loss is associated with all chronic disorders, e.g. chronic obstructive airways disease (COAD), chronic renal failure, and with malignancy in all sites. Undiagnosed poorly controlled diabetes mellitus and thyrotoxicosis and Addison's disease are other examples.

3 Psychiatric disease

The apathy of depression and the impaired insight and self-neglect in some demented patients will lead to attrition. The paranoia of a psychosis may make food unacceptable. The hyperactivity of some demented and hypomanic patients may result in weight loss. Alcohol abuse should also be considered.

4 Iatrogenic disease

Impaired appetite due to unpalatable treatment, e.g. spironolactone, or due to side effects caused by toxicity, e.g digoxin and L-Dopa, both potentially causing vomiting. Diarrhoea due to mefenamic acid and antibiotic treatment.

5 Gastrointestinal disease

- Dysphagia.
- Dyspepsia.
- Maldigestion.
- Malabsorption.

Dysphagia

1 Problems in mouth (see Chapter 19).
2 Neuromuscular causes.
3 Pressure on the oesophagus.
4 Narrowing due to change in the wall.
5 Epithelial causes.
6 Intraluminal obstruction.

Neuromuscular dysphagia

1 Ageing (presbyoesophagus). Uncoordinated oesophageal contractions or reduced activity. The smooth sequence of swallowing, i.e. rhythmic peristaltic contractions with relaxation of the cardia is lost or impaired. Best demonstrated by barium sandwich technique or isotope-transit time studies, or cineradiography.

2 Cerebrovascular disease. In hemiplegia with involvement of lower cranial nerves; more common and more severe in brain stem lesions, patients with bilateral hemisphere disease are especially at risk (pseudobulbar palsy).

3 Bulbar palsy, e.g. motor neurone disease.

4 Parkinson's disease. Akinesia complicates swallowing—may respond to L-dopa and speech therapy techniques. About 26 per cent of patients are affected. ANS dysfunction also common.

5 Myasthenia gravis. Rare but important because of good response to specific treatment with anticholinesterases.

6 Achalasia. More a problem of younger and middle-aged patients but may be an aspect of presbyoesophagus.
NB Nasogastric tube feeding usually only justified on a short-term basis when recovery can be reasonably expected. Narrow-gauged tubes should be used and only when the patient is aware of the problems and who, with help, will be able to cooperate in this form of management—especially if long-term treatment is contemplated.

Outside pressure on the oesophagus

1 Pharyngeal pouches. All pouches become more common with increasing age. Zenker's diverticulum through the posterior pharyngeal wall at the upper level of the cricopharyngeous may result from incoordinated contractions. When large and full may hinder normal passage down the oesophagus. X-ray diagnosis safest—endoscopy can be dangerous if lesion not suspected. Large and symptomatic pouches should be removed surgically. More rarely pouches may also occur at lower levels in the oesophagus.

2 Superior mediastinal obstruction. Secondary to malignancy (usually carcinoma of the bronchus) may be complicated by dysphagia.

3 Dilatation of the left atrium. Especially in mitral stenosis, can lead to dysphagia. A simple chest X-ray in conjunction with clinical signs will usually be sufficient to make the diagnosis.

4 Aortic arch dilatation.

Changes in the oesophageal wall

Carcinoma of the oesophagus is the most important diagnosis. Position can usually be well localized by the patient's symptoms which are likely to arise when two-thirds of the lumen is closed. Problems with solids, therefore, are the first and most important clue. X-ray is safest for diagnosis and great care is needed during endoscopy because of risk of perforation (results of X-ray examination should always be available prior to endoscopy). Endoscopy allows biopsy when the nature of the lesion is in doubt.

Treatment

Results are generally poor but palliation is valuable.

1 Surgery—for lesions at lower end.

2 Radiation—for lesions at the upper end.

3 Tube insertion—when other measures are unjustified; complications with this method are common and obstruction is likely to occur at a later date.

Inflammatory lesions of the epithelium

1 Oesophagitis—with or without stricture, usually at the lower end and associated with hiatus hernia and acid reflux, therefore long previous history may be given. Endoscopy is the best diagnostic approach and allows biopsy to be taken (essential if any suspicion of malignant change), and also enables recognition of Barret's oesophagus (gastric mucosa in the oesophagus).

Peptic oesophagitis should be treated with antacids or other simple remedies. H_2 antagonists will be needed in resistant cases and strictures should be dilated.

2 Oesophageal moniliasis—the frail elderly are at risk, especially those who have received antibiotics or are immunosuppressed. The typical white patches of thrush are often (but not always) present in the mouth. Endoscopy or barium swallow needed for confirmation of the oesophageal involvement.

Intraluminal obstruction
Impacted objects may include food residue, missing dentures and other foreign bodies. The demented are particularly at risk.

Dyspepsia

1 Indigestion is common at all ages (31 per cent of the population) and 2–3 per cent of prescribed drugs are antacids.
2 In many elderly patients their symptoms are very vague and non-specific and diagnosis, therefore, becomes increasingly difficult.
3 The potentially responsible lesions for indigestion become more common in old age, for example:
>   Hiatus hernia 60 per cent over 70 years of age
>   Peptic ulceration 20 per cent over 70 years of age
>   Gallstones 38 per cent over 70 years of age
>   Pancreatic disease
>   Mesenteric ischaemia
>   Carcinoma of large bowel
>   Carcinoma of stomach
>   Gastritis

4 Many of these conditions are asymptomatic, e.g. 21 per cent of hiatus hernia and up to 50 per cent of gallstones.
5 Many patients will have more than one possible cause for their non-specific indigestion—a therapeutic trial may be the only way of identifying the responsible lesion.
6 Endoscopy is a very acceptable form of investigation for most elderly patients and it is the investigation of first choice—care will be needed with premedication in those with poor respiratory reserve. ERCP is most helpful in elderly patients with biliary tract disease—and stones, if not too large, can be removed directly.
7 Ultrasound examination is the best technique for suspected gallbladder and pancreatic disease.
8 Special attention will be required when treatment is started, for example:
(i) Metoclopropamide—may precipitate or worsen extra pyramidal syndromes.

(ii) Cimetidine can cause confusion.

(iii) Aluminium salts should be avoided in constipated patients.

(iv) Carbonoxolone may cause serious hypokalaemia with life-threatening consequences in the frail elderly.

(v) Bile salts have proved disappointing for dissolving gallstones—side effects, especially diarrhoea, can be very troublesome in the elderly.

9 Many drugs cause dyspepsia, therefore drug history is a very important part of the investigation and assessment.

Gastrointestinal bleeding

1 Almost every recognized cause of gastrointestinal bleeding becomes more common with increasing age:

(i) Hiatus hernia with oesophagitis.

(ii) Gastritis—gastric erosions—elderly patients on non-steroidal anti-inflammatories have a sevenfold increased risk of bleeding compared with the same age group not taking such drugs.

(iii) Duodenal ulcer and gastric ulcer.

(iv) Carcinoma of the stomach (see Fig. 14.1).

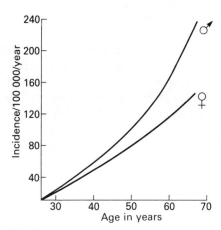

Special risk groups
(1) Old age — ×6 more common in old age v middle age
(2) Patients with PA — × 3–4 increased risk
(3) Previous gastric resection — ×5 increase
(4) Atrophic gastritis

Fig. 14.1. Carcinoma of the stomach.

(v) Diverticular disease.

(vi) Ischaemic bowel disease, sometimes difficult to differentiate from chronic inflammatory disease, e.g. Crohn's.

(vii) Carcinoma of the large bowel.

(viii) Piles.

(ix) Colonic polyps—40 per cent incidence in over 65 years in post-mortem study.

(x) Angiodysplasia of the colon.

Chronic blood loss—chronic gastrointestinal bleeding is the most common cause of iron deficiency anaemia in old age (see Chapter 17).

The bleeding site will be asymptomatic in many patients. Investigation is therefore problematic—examination of both the upper and lower tract will be required in many cases and the ready acceptance of a simple benign lesion should not prevent further exploration for more serious causes—if the patient is sufficiently fit and cooperative to undergo extensive examination.

Suggested plan of investigation:

(i) Confirmation of iron deficiency anaemia.

(ii) Confirmation of gastrointestinal bleeding—positive faecal occult bloods.

(iii) Endoscopy of upper tract—to reveal or exclude oesophagitis and gastritis, as well as definite ulceration and malignancy. Barium swallow/meal is more appropriate if dysphagia is a problem.

(iv) Sigmoidoscopy followed by barium enema to study large bowel—preferably as an inpatient in frail elderly patients to ensure adequate bowel preparation.

(v) Colonoscopy if barium enema is inconclusive—may confirm abnormality previously seen or reveal angiodysplasia.

(vi) Radio isotope labelled red cells may be used to confirm presence and site of gastrointestinal bleeding in difficult cases.

Treatment

(i) Specific treatment for underlying cause.

(ii) Oral iron supplements—ferrous sulphate if tolerated.

(iii) Transfuse only if haemoglobin is very low, e.g. less than 7 g and patient unwell; take care if risk of congestive heart failure present.

Acute blood loss
Particularly dangerous in the elderly as the resulting hypotension
may trigger off pathological changes in other systems, e.g. stroke,
myocardial infarction and renal failure. Speedy treatment is
therefore required, initially blood transfusion but with quick and
ready access to surgical intervention if the bleeding persists.

Even very acute upper gastrointestinal bleeding in the elderly
can present as melaena rather than haematemesis—endoscopy may
therefore be helpful in locating the site of bleeding.

Acute and severe ischaemia may present as rectal bleeding—
but the ischaemia may be secondary to other pathology, e.g. a silent
myocardial infarction—a full assessment is therefore needed.

The acute abdomen

A difficult diagnostic problem at all ages, but even more so in old
age. The mortality rate in elderly patients is much higher and may
exceed 50 per cent in some instances; there are 4 possible reasons
for such depressing results:
1 Delay in presentation.
2 Atypical presentation ('silent').
3 Reluctance to operate on frail elderly patients.
4 Precipitation of other significant pathology during the acute
episode, e.g. myocardial infarction and stroke.

For pathology found in patients over 75 years undergoing
emergency abdominal surgery see Table 14.1.

Table 14.1.

Diagnosis	Number	Mortality rate (%)
Strangulated hernia	115	16.5
Intestinal obstruction	103	37.9
Perforated peptic ulcer	22	40.9
Perforated large bowel	22	63.6
Ruptured aortic aneurysm	9	77.7
Biliary tract disease*	22	
Mesenteric ischaemia*	10	

*Reduced numbers as some patients were treated conservatively

Useful investigations in the elderly acute abdomen:
1 Check hernial orifices.
2 X-ray for fluid levels.
3 X-ray for free air in peritoneal cavity.
4 Check amylase level—about half the patients with acute pancreatitis are over 60 years of age.
5 Use ultrasound for detection of aortic aneurysm and monitor presence of pulses.

NB Always consider the diagnosis of 'acute abdomen' in 'shocked', elderly patients, if supporting evidence is found on examination and emergency investigation, act quickly if surgical help is indicated.

Bowel ischaemia

1 Twenty per cent of cardiac output is used to supply the gastrointestinal tract—the cerebral circulation is normally protected from sudden decreases in supply, therefore any significant change in cardiac output is likely to affect the perfusion of the bowel permitting ischaemia to occur.
2 At least 2 major mesenteric arteries must be compromised for bowel ischaemia to occur.
3 Because of a poor anastomotic arrangement, the left side of the colon is the most vulnerable segment of the bowel.

Clinical course

1 Mild
(i) Abdominal pain plus blood loss.
(ii) Mucosal swelling–thumb printing on barium studies.
(iii) Recovery plus or minus scarring (stricture).

2 Severe
(i) Sudden severe pain.
(ii) Movement of fluid into lumen, vomiting, diarrhoea and shock.
(iii) Ischaemic bowel wall allows bacteria to cross from lumen to peritoneum—peritonitis plus or minus septicaemia.
(iv) Death almost certain.

Treatment
Acute/mild—support and treat underlying cause to prevent recurrence.

Acute/severe—consult surgeons regarding resection; supportive and symptomatic treatment.

Chronic—small frequent meals; correct any nutritional deficiencies due to malabsorption.

Diarrhoea

A very incapacitating condition in old age, especially if the patient is already disabled and immobile due to other pathologies.

1 Spurious, i.e. obstruction with overflow must be excluded first by rectal examination with or without sigmoidoscopy. The cause may be simple, e.g. faecal impaction, or serious, e.g. carcinoma of the rectum.

2 Infective—cultures must be taken and patient isolated whilst results awaited:

(i) Viral—most common, usually self-limiting and supportive measures only required.

(ii) Bacterial—antibiotics only justified if patient's condition is grave, in mild cases they may prolong symptoms.

(iii) Chronic bowel infection—may be endemic in institutions (e.g. *Clostridium difficile*).

3 Inflammatory—Crohn's disease of large bowel most common, chronic inflammatory bowel disease in old age; diagnosis by biopsy and barium studies.

4 Metabolic—uncommon but exclude thyrotoxicosis; some cases secondary to diabetic neuropathy.

5 Iatrogenic—antibiotic diarrhoea common; purgative misuse; gastrectomy/vagotomy.

Constipation

Fear of becoming constipated is more an aspect of old age than a genuine symptom. Seventy-one per cent of elderly people have their bowels open once daily, 11 per cent every other day and 14 per cent twice daily. Causes are:

(i) Faulty habits—low residue diet, low fluid intake, lack of exercise and neglect of call to stool.

(ii) Poor appetite.

(iii) Immobility.

(iv) Drugs—analgesics, anticholinergics and diuretics.

(v) Metabolic—myxoedema, hypercalcaemia.

(vi) Psychiatric—depression, dementia.
(vii) Functional—irritable bowel, purgative abuse (cathartic colon).
(viii) Pain—piles and fissures.

Change in bowel habit

Alternating diarrhoea and constipation always a worrying symptom. Carcinoma of the large bowel must be excluded but diverticular disease or large bowel ischaemia and irritable colon are more common.

Barium enema examination can be an ordeal in frail elderly patients. Best results are obtained if the patient is admitted for good bowel preparation and sigmoidoscopy before the procedure.

Faecal incontinence

1 Spurious diarrhoea due to faecal impaction (sometimes beyond rectal examination) is commonest cause, especially in demented patients.
2 Circumstantial, i.e. intestinal hurry plus physical immobility equals faecal incontinence. Treat underlying causes and reduce distance to toilet or commode.
3 Neurological or structural, e.g. paraplegia or rectal prolapse. Treat underlying cause where possible, e.g. surgery for rectal prolapse. If cure impossible—cause constipation with codeine phosphate and bulking preparations and relieve bowels at regular intervals with enemata.
4 Inhibition and lack of insight, e.g. in dementia. Bulking preparation and encourage regular toileting habits and facilitate recognition of toilet (e.g. large visible signs or brightly coloured lavatory door); protective clothing if all else fails.

Absorption

1 Small bowel function declines with age but nutritional deficiencies only occur when additional factors intervene, e.g. poor diet or ill health.
2 Causes of malabsorption in youth may also occur *de novo* in old age, e.g. adult coeliac disease.

3 Maldigestion is more common than malabsorption, e.g. due to pancreatic disease.

4 Bacterial change in the small bowel lumen due to stasis or diverticular disease is common (10 per cent of elderly people) and is frequently clinically significant.

5 Ischaemia is a special cause of malabsorption in old age.

6 Iatrogenic causes must always be considered, e.g. postgastrectomy, alcohol and some drugs, e.g. biguanides and oral neomycin.

Possible indicators of malabsorption

1 Weight loss in spite of good dietary intake.

2 Low serum albumin level.

3 Unexplained iron deficiency anaemia (with negative faecal occult bloods).

4 Macrocytic anaemia.

5 Osteomalacia.

Potential causes of malabsorption in old age

The investigation of malabsorption in old age is very difficult and unsatisfactory but the following possibilities should always be considered and explored wherever possible:

1 Previous gastrectomy.

2 Small bowel diverticular disease.

3 Altered luminal bacterial flora.

4 Pancreatic disease—causes maldigestion.

5 Adult coeliac disease.

6 Lymphoma.

7 Crohn's disease.

8 Mesenteric ischaemia.

9 Folate deficiency, C_2H_5OH abuse.

10 Drugs, e.g. neomycin, biguanides, cholestyramine.

Jaundice

Surgical causes are common and must be identified rapidly before the patient becomes irremediable—ultrasound examination is the investigation of first choice. Medical causes of jaundice should be investigated and treated as in younger patients.

Non-invasive techniques of value in elderly patients with biliary disease

1 Dissolving gallstones—radiotranslucent stones only and in the absence of biliary obstruction chenodeoxycholic acid may be used but diarrhoea can be an important side effect. Prolonged treatment (over 2 years) may be required; stones may recur.
2 Sphincterotomy—during ERCP will allow obstructing stones to escape.
3 Stent insertion—during ERCP may relieve obstruction caused by carcinoma of the pancreas or cholangiocarcinoma.

Further reading

Coakley D. (ed.) (1981) Gastrointestinal emergencies in the elderly. In: James O. *Acute Geriatric Medicine*. Croom Helm, London.
Hellemans J. & Vantrappen G. (eds.) (1984) *Gastrointestinal Disorder in the Elderly*. Churchill Livingstone, Edinburgh.

Chapter 15
Homeostatic Failure
(Metabolic and Endocrine Disorders)

Age changes

1 Lean body mass and body water are reduced; there is usually an increase in fat.

2 Endocrine changes are as follows:

- Serum levels of noradrenaline ↑.
- Serum levels of renin, aldosterone ↓.
- Heart less responsive to beta–adrenergic stimulation.
- Carbohydrate tolerance deteriorates.
- Serum ADH ↑ (but renal response ↓).
- Oestrogen falls to 20 per cent premenopausal value.
- Testosterone levels unchanged in female, ↓ in male.
- FSH and LH levels ↑.
- Adenomas common in anterior pituitary, thyroid and adrenal.

Disorders of fluid and electrolyte balance

Fluid loss and overload

Both dehydration and oedema are very common in the old. Some reasons for the former are listed below and causes of the latter are given in Table 15.1. Paradoxically, the two may coexist in the 'top and bottom' syndrome of puffy ankles and diminished tissue turgor in the upper extremities together with a low circulating volume. To observe a little swelling of the feet should not necessarily lead to prescribing a diuretic, but if one is prescribed, it must not be assumed that it is on a long-term basis.

Where dehydration is due to mixed salt and water depletion (as in gastrointestinal or renal loss), the extracellular fluid (ECF) is mainly affected leading to poor tissue turgor, postural hypotension, tachycardia and relative polycythaemia. Where it is mainly due to water depletion caused by an inadequate intake, the intracellular fluid (ICF) bears the brunt. Various studies have shown that the normal thirst mechanism is often deficient in these subjects and that

Table 15.1. Common causes of oedema

Fluid retention	1 Drugs
	2 Cardiac failure
	3 Renal failure
Raised venous pressure	1 Cardiac failure
	2 Venous insufficiency or thrombosis
	3 Lack of muscle pump action (prolonged sitting)
Hypoalbuminaemia	1 Malnutrition, liver disease
	2 Protein loss
Lymphatic obstruction	Usually malignant
Capillary wall defect	Inflammatory—e.g. cellulitis

the tubular capacity to respond to Antidiuretic hormone (ADH) is often defective although ADH output is adequate. Confusion and weakness are characteristic of both types of dehydration.

Reasons for vulnerability of the aged to dehydration

1 Reduction in body water.
2 Reluctance to drink through fear of incontinence, nocturnal frequency, or being caught short while out and about.
3 Lack of motivation or ability to drink sufficiently due to ill-health, depression, immobility.
4 Widespread diuretic misuse.
5 Prevalence of dehydrating disease (swallowing disorders, diabetes, purgative abuse).
6 Impaired concentrating ability of kidney and diminished renal response to ADH.
7 Defective osmoregulatory function impairs thirst response.

Hyponatraemia

This is a particularly common phenomenon in geriatric practice and can be classified as in Fig. 15.1. A contributory factor may be a very low salt intake for some time prior to estimation.

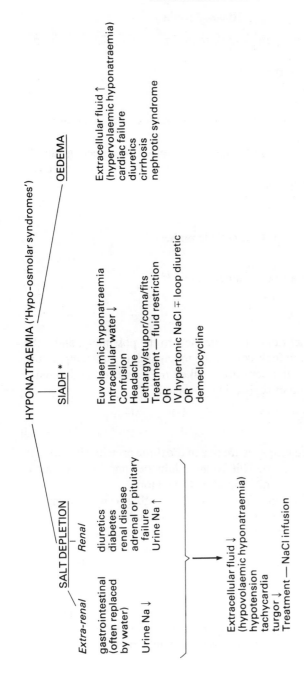

HYPONATRAEMIA ('Hypo-osmolar syndromes')

SALT DEPLETION

Extra-renal

gastrointestinal
(often replaced
by water)

Urine Na ↓

Renal

diuretics
diabetes
renal disease
adrenal or pituitary
failure
Urine Na ↑

Extracellular fluid ↓
(hypovolaemic hyponatraemia)
hypotension
tachycardia
turgor ↓
Treatment — NaCl infusion

SIADH *

Euvolaemic hyponatraemia
Intracellular water ↓
Confusion
Headache
Lethargy/stupor/coma/fits
Treatment — fluid restriction
OR
IV hypertonic NaCl ∓ loop diuretic
OR
demeclocycline

OEDEMA

Extracellular fluid ↑
(hypervolaemic hyponatraemia)
cardiac failure
diuretics
cirrhosis
nephrotic syndrome

* SIADH = Syndrome of inappropriate ADH secretion
Diagnostic criteria include hypo-osmolar plasma, urine of high osmolality,
no evidence of hypovolaemia or drugs or other disease states, and good response to correction

Fig. 15.1. Classification of hyponatraemia.

Hypokalaemia

Hypokalaemia is again widespread among the sick old for the following reasons:
- Inadequate dietary intake.
- Gastrointestinal loss.
- Diuretic therapy.
- Cushing's syndrome, commonly iatrogenic or due to carcinoma of bronchus.
- 'Acute transient hypokalaemia', reported as affecting elderly females with systemic illness, self-correcting in about 4 days, possibly caused by shift into cells.

Accidental hypothermia

Definition
The core temperature has fallen below 35°C.

Diagnosis
The general practitioner must be alert to the possibility, and if the patient's abdomen feels cold to the touch and the oral temperature is low, the rectal temperature is taken over a period of 5 minutes using a thermometer registering down to 25°C.

Aetiology
See Fig. 15.2; the more severe one of the three principal factors, the less the others need be. Fit young adults become hypothermic if their yachts capsize while rounding Cape Horn.

It has been found that aged subjects liable to hypothermia in conditions which are not unduly severe are unable to maintain an adequate core/periphery gradient, and that shivering during cooling occurs in far fewer elderly than young subjects. The vasoconstrictor response to cooling is often virtually absent, and conversely, sweating on rewarming is often absent or requires a greater temperature rise to initiate it. These mechanisms are mediated by the autonomic nervous system (ANS; Chapter 11). Finally, temperature discrimination has been shown to be less sensitive in older subjects compared to younger ones.

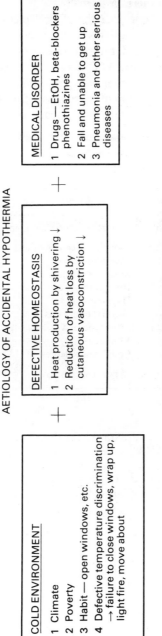

AETIOLOGY OF ACCIDENTAL HYPOTHERMIA

COLD ENVIRONMENT

1 Climate
2 Poverty
3 Habit — open windows, etc.
4 Defective temperature discrimination
   → failure to close windows, wrap up,
   light fire, move about

+

DEFECTIVE HOMEOSTASIS

1 Heat production by shivering ↓
2 Reduction of heat loss by
   cutaneous vasoconstriction ↓

+

MEDICAL DISORDER

1 Drugs — EtOH, beta-blockers
   phenothiazines
2 Fall and unable to get up
3 Pneumonia and other serious
   diseases

= HYPOTHERMIA

Fig. 15.2.

Clinical features of hypothermia
As will be seen from Table 15.2 the clinical picture may closely mimic hypothyroidism although this is the cause in a small minority of cases. When the core temperature is over 30°C, the mortality is about 33 per cent, but below 30°C it rises to 70 per cent. These figures reflect not only the danger of hypothermia itself but also the extremely precarious condition of those most often affected. Complications include pancreatitis, hypoglycaemia and ventricular arrhythmias.

Table 15.2. Hypothermia

Core temperature	Clinical feature
32–35°C	May be few other than 'going off'
< 32°C	Clouding of consciousness, sluggishness
	Muscular rigidity
	Bradycardia
	Hypotension
	Oliguria or diuresis
	J waves on ECG
	Vomiting
	Cough reflex depressed
< 27°C	75 per cent comatose

Management of hypothermia

(a) Mild cases, temperature 34°C
Wrap up warmly, give hot drink, switch on electric fire, close window, counsel to prevent recurrence.

(b) Temperature over 32°C
Cautious passive rewarming at 0.5–1°C per hour to avoid catastrophic hypotension, use metallized reflective blanket and minimal intervention; treat concomitant illness.

(c) *Temperature below 30°C*
The statistics are so abysmal that the following high risk, aggressive

measures have been increasingly recommended:
(i) Active rewarming by IV fluids or gastric lavage or colonic lavage or peritoneal lavage (> 38°C).
(ii) Ventilate if necessary.
(iii) ECG monitoring.
(iv) CVP monitoring.
(v) IV antibiotics.
(vi) Monitor rectal temperature, BP, blood gases.
(vii) Monitor glucose and electrolytes.
(viii) Treat concomitant disease.

Prevention of hypothermia
Common sense indicates the appropriate advice except that lay persons will not realize that up to half the body's heat is lost through the scalp. A useful Christmas present is therefore a woolly nightcap. An alternative suggestion is an easy-to-read wall thermometer. It is also important to keep in mind those at special risk, especially during cold spells.

High risk groups
1 Patients with systemic illness.
2 The demented and the depressed.
3 The poor and the inadequately housed.
4 Those prone to falls.
5 Patients with ANS dysfunction.
6 Patients on the drugs mentioned.
7 The malnourished are especially prone to rapid cooling.

Other hazards of winter

In an average winter in England and Wales there are about 40000 deaths in excess of those to be expected during this period of time, mainly due to stroke and myocardial infarction. This may be related to increases in platelets, haematocrit, blood viscosity, and plasma cholesterol on exposure to the cold. The BP also shows a marked variation with environmental temperature, the SBP in older men in particular rising when it is cold. Falling on icy pavements may be an additional minor contributory factor to this excess mortality.

Heat illness

Although cerebrovascular accidents and mortality rates have been shown to increase among the aged in the UK during heat waves, heat illness has not been shown to occur. It does in hotter climates, however, due to impairment of temperature control.

Diabetes mellitus

Definition

See Table 15.3. A raised haemoglobin AIC level can give an indication of persistent hyperglycaemia during the preceding 2 to 6 weeks.

Table 15.3. Definition of diabetes

	mmol/l	mg/100 ml
1 Fasting bs [1]	8	144
+symptoms *or* random bs	11	198
2 2-hour GTT [2] bs	11	198
3 'Impaired glucose tolerance'		
fasting bs	8	144
2-hour GTT bs	8–11	144–198
4 Diabetes *excluded*		
fasting bs	6	108
random bs	8	144
2-hour GTT bs	6.7	

1. bs = venous blood sugar.
2. GTT = glucose tolerance test using 75 g anhydrous glucose taken orally.
(Source: World Health Organization, 1980: WHO Expert Committee on Diabetes Mellitus. Technical Report Series 646: WHO, Geneva.) Note: Other commonly used upper limits of normal include a random bs of 10 mmol/l (180 mg/100 ml), a fasting bs 7.2 mmol/l (130 mg/100 ml) and a 2-hour GTT bs of 12.2 mmol/l (220 mg/100 ml).

Glucose tolerance declines with advancing age, but most cases of diabetes are of the non-insulin dependent diabetes mellitus (NIDDM) type which is less prone to ketoacidosis and in which there is delayed insulin secretion in response to a glucose load and a

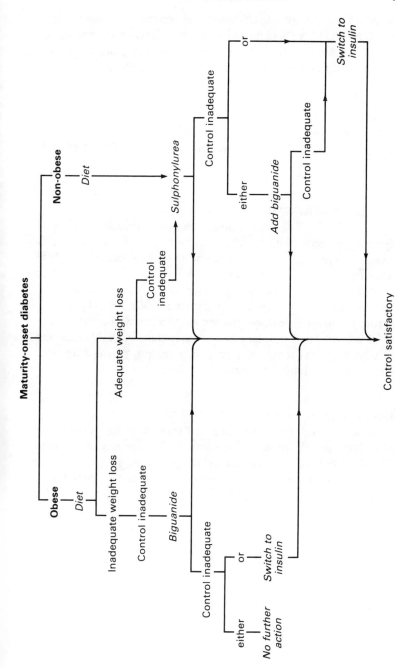

Fig. 15.3. Flow chart for treatment of diabetes.

degree of insulin resistance due to a receptor or post-receptor defect. NIDDM is also known as type II, and was formerly termed maturity onset diabetes. A small proportion of elderly diabetics require insulin, either long term or during acute illnesses.

Incidence
Over the age of 70, 20 per cent of men and 30 per cent of women show an abnormality of glucose tolerance generally regarded as diabetic.

Management of NIDDM
See Fig. 15.3. The aim should be to maintain reasonably physiological blood sugar levels in patients in their sixties or early seventies to avoid or delay complications. In patients in their late seventies or eighties, a more reasonable ambition is freedom from symptoms and, at least as important, the avoidance of hypoglycaemia. This is because of the vulnerability of old people to neuronal damage from hypoglycaemia, which may take the form of confusion, fits, or focal deficits such as hemiparesis. Atypical and resistant hypoglycaemia is a particular feature of sulphonylurea treatment, especially the longacting varieties.

Diabetic crises
Ketoacidosis and hypoglycaemia are treated along conventional lines. The complication which seems to be virtually confined to NIDDM is hyperosmolar coma and the preceding diabetic state has often been mild and easily controlled. It is due to progressive dehydration on account of an osmotic diuresis, and the onset is insidious with eventual clouding of consciousness or coma. Hypotension is a frequent finding and extreme hyperglycaemia is typically accompanied by hypernatraemia and uraemia. Half normal saline is infused at a rate of 0.5 litres per hour and up to 10 litres of fluid over and above the output may be required in the first 48 hours or so; ideally the central venous pressure should be monitored. The initial dose of insulin is usually 20 units iv or im followed by 5 units subcutaneously hourly or two hourly. The mortality is high, but survivors are often discharged on diet alone or oral therapy.

Thyrotoxicosis

This disease differs clinically from Grave's disease (Table 15.4).

Table 15.4. Distinguishing features of hyperthyroidism in old age

Feature	Younger patients	Older patients
Goitre	Diffuse	Nodular or absent
Eye signs	Often prominent	Seldom prominent
Pulse	Sinus tachycardia	Atrial fibrillation
Heart failure	Rare	Common
Hot, sweaty hands	Common	Uncommon
Tremor	Fine	Atypical or absent
Weakness and wasting	Not striking	Often dominant feature
Irritability, hyperkinesis	Often marked	Seldom marked
Gastrointestinal	Increased appetite, loose bowels	Not typical

Diagnosis
Clinical diagnosis is therefore often very difficult, and the question arises whether tests of thyroid function should be performed routinely on every elderly patient with atrial fibrillation, or admitted to a medical/geriatric ward, or seen by the GP. This question has not been resolved, but it is at least clear that newer, more refined techniques for the assay of thyrotropin (TSH) offer the best single test of thyroid function, since low levels indicative of hyperthyroidism can now be measured with accuracy.

Treatment
(a) Very rapid effect desired; carbimazole plus beta-adrenoceptor blocking drug until ventricular rate responds.

(b) Rapid effect desired; carbimazole until satisfactory response followed by radio-iodine. The carbimazole is withdrawn 48 hours prior to radio-iodine and can be started 48 hours after the dose and then gradually tailed off.

(c) No urgency; proceed directly to radio-iodine. A response occurs after 2 to 3 months. Prolonged follow-up is necessary in all cases to detect recurrence and hypothyroidism.

Hypothyroidism

The classic features of this disease are well known but atypical cases are sufficiently common for only a minority of patients to be recognized without resort to the use of serum T_4 and TSH levels as a screening procedure. It is usual to give replacement therapy on a once daily basis, but it should be started with extreme caution. The initial dose is 25 mcg daily and increments of 25 mcg added every 2 weeks until the correct dose is achieved as reflected by the clinical state and the TSH level. The usual total daily requirement is not more than 150 mcg in older people.

Hypopituitarism

Idiopathic pituitary failure is only mentioned because of recent reports drawing attention to numbers of aged patients detected during episodes of systemic illness in which the appearance, a low plasma sodium level and orthostatic hypotension were among the clinical features. We ourselves have some evidence that the condition may be commoner than suspected.

Addison's disease

This uncommon condition may be due to tuberculosis, carcinomatosis, or auto-immune atrophy. It is mentioned since it may be a cause of 'failure to thrive' and also because it may present as a crisis, often due to injudicious cessation of corticosteroid therapy or intercurrent illness in a patient whose steroids have recently been reduced or withdrawn.

Further reading

Anon (1984) Thirst and osmoregulation in the elderly. *Lancet,* **ii,** 1017–18.

Emslie–Smith D. (1981) Hypothermia in the elderly. *British Journal of Hospital Medicine,* **26,** 442–52.

Flear C.T.G., Gill G.V. & Burn J. (1981) Hyponatraemia: mechanisms and management. *Lancet,* **ii,** 26–31.

Keatinge W. (1986) Medical problems of cold weather. *Journal of the Royal College of Physicians of London,* **20,** 283–7.

Wright A.D. & Kilvert A. (1985) Diabetes mellitus. In: Isaacs, B. (ed.) *Recent Advances in Geriatric Medicine,* Vol. 3, pp. 1–17. Churchill Livingstone, Edinburgh.

Chapter 16
Urogenital System

Ageing changes

1 In old age renal function is reduced to about 50 per cent of peak function (i.e. that at age of 30 years).

2 The blood urea in healthy old age remains normal in spite of falling renal function.

3 The aged kidney has impaired ability to both concentrate urine and to process an extra water load.

4 Renal scarring is evident in 46 per cent of 'normal' elderly kidneys.

5 Falling renal function is due to:

(i) Nephron 'drop out'.

(ii) Vascular changes.

(iii) Poor response to ADH.

6 The combination of renal ageing changes and systemic or renal disease may lead to rapid and dramatic renal failure in elderly patients.

7 Atrophic changes occur in the urogenital tract of postmenopausal women.

8 Prostatic size increases with age.

9 The unstable bladder with detrusor instability becomes increasingly common in old age but bladder control is only likely to be lost when aggravating factors also occur (see Table 16.1).

Table 16.1. Detrusor instability—exacerbating factors

Environmental
Mobility
UTI (urinary tract infection)
Vaginitis
Diuretics
Diabetes
Tranquillizers/hypnotics

Renal failure in old age

Pre-renal and post-renal causes are most frequently responsible. Patients must therefore be rehydrated and renal tract obstruction must be excluded (by clinical examination and ultrasound)—on presentation. Intrinsic renal disease (except infection) is not often of paramount clinical importance in geriatric patients and age alone should not be used as a contraindication for renal dialysis.

Infection

Urinary tract infections (bacteriuria greater than 10^5) are common in old age. Twenty per cent of people over the age of 65 will experience a urinary tract infection. Pyelonephritis is responsible for 20 per cent of cases of renal failure. Precipitating factors for urinary tract infections in old age:

(i) High incidence of urinary stasis—poor bladder emptying
prostatism
diverticula.

(ii) Hormonal changes affecting the mucous membranes of women.

(iii) Associated disorders—diabetes
atherosclerosis
immobility
indwelling catheter.

(iv) Stones.

Unusual presentations of urinary tract infection in old age

(i) Asymptomatic i.e. found on screening—should remain untreated if patient is well.

(ii) Acute toxic state—catheterization may be required to obtain specimen, alternatively organism may on some occasions be obtained on blood culture.

(iii) Onset of incontinence.

(iv) Increasing drowsiness due to worsening renal failure.

Management

(i) Attempt to obtain organism from urine or blood.

(ii) Maintain good fluid input (greater than 2 litres per day).

(iii) Give appropriate antibiotics (trimethoprim best 'blind treatment').

(iv) Reverse precipitating cause, if possible (see Section 3 above).

Obstructive nephropathy

1 Lesion in urethra
(i) Males.

(ii) Past history of previous episodes of venereal disease.

(iii) Bladder palpable or demonstrable on ultrasound.

(iv) Catheterization difficult or impossible, expert help will be needed.

2 Bladder neck obstruction

A Prostate pathology

(i) By the eighth decade 50 per cent of prostates contain areas of benign nodular hyperplasia, chronic prostatitis, pre-malignant changes.

(ii) Less than half of men with benign prostatic hypertrophy develop symptoms of obstruction.

(iii) Only 1 per cent of prostatic cancers cause problems during life, but clinically second most frequent malignancy in men.

(iv) Rectal examination first essential step in diagnosis.

(v) Biopsy of suspicious nodules—?carcinoma.

(vi) Raised acid phosphatase levels support diagnosis of carcinoma.

(vii) Treatment of benign hypertrophy—transurethral prostatectomy—(TURP).

(viii) Treatment of carcinoma (orchidectomy or hormone therapy) depending on spread and patient's preferences.

(ix) Chance finding of malignant specimen in TURP specimen, management remains problematic, many patients will live trouble free (see Chapter 18 and Fig. 16.1).

B Gynaecological problems—detectable on pelvic examination
(i) Malignancy of female genital tract.

(ii) Hormone deficient changes in mucosa of trigone of bladder.

C Spread of rectal malignancy—detectable on rectal examination and on CT scanning.

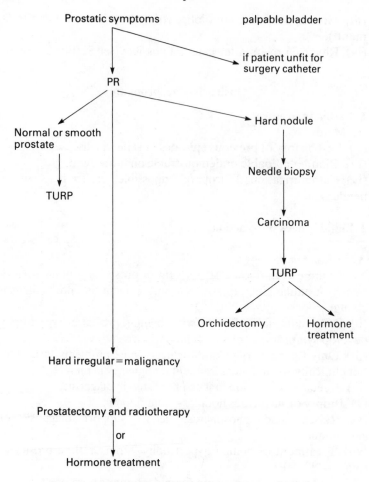

Fig. 16.1. Management of patients with prostatic symptoms.

D Faecal impaction—must always be excluded.

E Neurological disease—affecting bladder emptying.

3 Retroperitoneal disease—malignancy and fibrosis (latter may be drug induced, e.g. by beta-blockers and methysergide).

4 Unilateral disease—due to ureteric obstruction, secondary to stones, malignancy or fibrosis.

Drugs and the kidneys

1 Nephrotoxic drugs.
(i) Antibiotics, e.g. streptomycin, gentamycin and tetracycline.
(ii) Analgesics, e.g. non-steroidal anti-inflammatories, phenacetin.
(iii) Antirheumatics, e.g. penacilliamine, gold.
2 Overdosage of drugs acting on kidneys, i.e. diuretics leading to dehydration, hypotension and electrolyte imbalance and to the extent of causing marked renal failure.
3 Renal changes causing drug toxicity, i.e. in drugs excreted via the kidneys—best example is digoxin.

Blood pressure and the kidneys

1 Renal disease may cause hypertension, e.g. chronic pyelon-ephritis.
2 The overtreatment of high blood pressure will impair renal function. Yet untreated hypertension may result in renal failure!
3 Hypotension, e.g. after bleeding, myocardial infarction or pulmonary embolus may result in renal shutdown and acute renal failure especially where renal function is already compromised by extreme old age or pathological changes.

Haematuria

1 Contamination, e.g. vaginal bleeding.
2 Iatrogenic, e.g. anticoagulants.
3 Haematological disease—bleeding/clotting disorders.
4 Infective, including tuberculous infection.
5 Malignant—ultrasound of bladder is a helpful and non-invasive test but cystoscopy will be needed to obtain biopsies. Bleeding from higher points in renal tract will need investigation by urologists/radiologists; cytology of urine also helpful.
6 Stones.
7 Immune cause, i.e. microscopic haematuria, e.g. SBE, poly-arteritis nodosa.

4 There is an age-related increase in the incidence of auto-antibodies and the female preponderance is lost.

The erythrocyte sedimentation rate (ESR)

1 Moderately raised levels, e.g. 30 mm/h Westergren, are not uncommon even in the absence of manifest disease. This may represent occult disease rather than a phenomenon of ageing. Most healthy old people have a lower level than this.

2 Higher ESRs must be regarded as pathological although the pathology can elude detection despite a careful search for malignancy, renal tract disease, myelomatosis, connective tissue disorder, chronic infection and so forth. Such cases can be followed up for years without a serious illness developing. It has been suggested that some of these enigmas are *formes frustes* of myelomatosis.

3 Very low ESRs are seen in association with polycythaemia, congestive cardiac failure, anti-inflammatory drugs, cachexia and hyperproteinaemia with hyperviscosity.

4 C–reactive protein (CPR), an acute phase protein, is a more sensitive indicator of an inflammatory response than the ESR.

5 Although not so readily available, the plasma viscosity can be a more reliable guide to the presence of organic disease in elderly people. A raised level indicates disease and a low level suggests reduced plasma proteins.

Iron metabolism

1 Normal old people on a normal diet have no impairment of iron metabolism.

2 A dietary intake of 10 mg of iron daily allows a good margin of safety in both sexes (see also below).

3 Iron absorption usually is increased when iron stores are depleted but paradoxically may occasionally be reduced and improve with iron replacement. Absorption is also increased during phases of active erythropoiesis.

4 Plasma iron may be reduced by conditions other than iron deficiency, e.g. infection, malignancy and renal failure. Plasma iron and total iron binding capacity (TIBC) or transferrin level fall with age after the third and sixth decades respectively.

5 Serum ferritin tends to increase with age but nevertheless gives a reasonable approximation of the amount of stainable marrow iron. Ferritin and haemosiderin are the main storage forms.

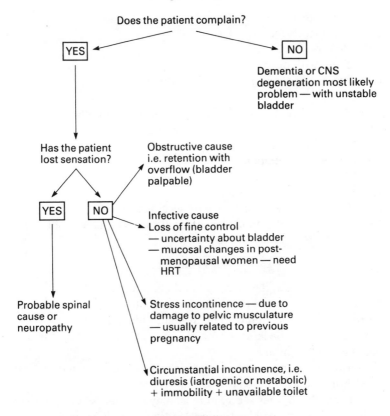

Fig. 16.2. Incontinence.

2 Examination
?Bladder palpable
PR ?prostate abnormal ?faecal impaction
PV evidence of senile vaginitis
CNS cord lesion or peripheral neuropathy
Mental test score—evidence of intellectual failure.

3 Investigations
Urinalysis—?glycosuria
MSU ?urinary infection
Urodynamic studies—mainly for research.

4 Therapeutic trial
(i) Clear infection.
(ii) Clear rectum.
(iii) Treat with oestrogens.
(iv) Pessary or repair for stress incontinence.
(v) TURP.
(vi) Reduce bladder activity, e.g. with anti-cholinergics.

5 In irreversible incontinence
(i) Supply pads and pants.
(ii) Make continence easier—plentiful and accessible toilets, regular toileting, obvious toilets.
(iii) Try appliances—usually only successful in men.
(iv) If patient understands and consents, use permanent catheter.

Sex in old age

1 Sexual activity and enjoyment may continue until the end of life.
2 Impotence becomes more common—but is not universal and is more usually associated with neurological impairment.
3 Erections may be less well maintained but premature ejaculation becomes uncommon.
4 Hormonal changes in the female urogenital tract may require that lubricants should be used to facilitate intercourse.
5 Physical disabilities—e.g. in hips, may prevent penetration—in which case other sexual activities ('petting') should be explored.
6 Sexual activity with a familiar partner is unlikely to cause sufficient excitement to precipitate fatal consequences (even in the presence of severe disease).
7 Disinhibited behaviour can be a serious problem in the management of elderly patients with widespread cerebral disease; considerable tolerance in the carers will be required.

Further reading

Brocklehurst J.C. (ed.) (1984) *Urology in the Elderly*. Churchill Livingstone, Edinburgh.

Chapter 17
Blood Diseases

Age changes

Red blood cells (RBC)
There is evidence of reduced deformability in health and this is even more marked in those with cerebrovascular disease.

White blood cells (WBC)
1 In elderly people more marked granulation (probably lysosymes) and lobulation of granulocytes has been described.
2 There is a tendency towards leucopenia with a normal leucocyte count range of $3-8.5 \times 10^9/l$ in old age.
3 The lymph nodes, the lymphoid tissue of the gastrointestinal tract and the spleen are all much reduced. The thymus is atrophied by middle age but thymic remnants are thought to remain active in extreme old age.
4 The B−cell population is well maintained but there is a reduction in T−cell numbers and functional capacity.
5 Some impairment of phagocytosis by neutrophils and macrophages has been reported.

Plasma proteins
Conflicting reports on age changes relate to the difficulty in separating those changes due solely to age and those due to other factors such as malnutrition or disease. The main points to emerge are:
1 Low levels of total protein and of the individual fractions are to be regarded as pathological.
2 Increased globulin fractions indicate disease and asymptomatic individuals with very high levels of gamma-globulin may have *formes frustes* of myelomatosis.
3 Abnormal immunoglobulins are increasingly common in the very old, being present in some 3 per cent of those aged over 70 years and in 20 per cent of those over 90.

4 There is an age-related increase in the incidence of auto-antibodies and the female preponderance is lost.

The erythrocyte sedimentation rate (ESR)

1 Moderately raised levels, e.g. 30 mm/h Westergren, are not uncommon even in the absence of manifest disease. This may represent occult disease rather than a phenomenon of ageing. Most healthy old people have a lower level than this.

2 Higher ESRs must be regarded as pathological although the pathology can elude detection despite a careful search for malignancy, renal tract disease, myelomatosis, connective tissue disorder, chronic infection and so forth. Such cases can be followed up for years without a serious illness developing. It has been suggested that some of these enigmas are *formes frustes* of myelomatosis.

3 Very low ESRs are seen in association with polycythaemia, congestive cardiac failure, anti-inflammatory drugs, cachexia and hyperproteinaemia with hyperviscosity.

4 C–reactive protein (CPR), an acute phase protein, is a more sensitive indicator of an inflammatory response than the ESR.

5 Although not so readily available, the plasma viscosity can be a more reliable guide to the presence of organic disease in elderly people. A raised level indicates disease and a low level suggests reduced plasma proteins.

Iron metabolism

1 Normal old people on a normal diet have no impairment of iron metabolism.

2 A dietary intake of 10 mg of iron daily allows a good margin of safety in both sexes (see also below).

3 Iron absorption usually is increased when iron stores are depleted but paradoxically may occasionally be reduced and improve with iron replacement. Absorption is also increased during phases of active erythropoiesis.

4 Plasma iron may be reduced by conditions other than iron deficiency, e.g. infection, malignancy and renal failure. Plasma iron and total iron binding capacity (TIBC) or transferrin level fall with age after the third and sixth decades respectively.

5 Serum ferritin tends to increase with age but nevertheless gives a reasonable approximation of the amount of stainable marrow iron. Ferritin and haemosiderin are the main storage forms.

6 Defective utilization of iron may be due to deficient transferrin levels as when protein synthesis is impaired, e.g. in gastrointestinal or renal disease. A similar mechanism may be operative in other chronic illness such as infection, connective tissue disease and malignancy.

Haemopoiesis and ageing

1 There is a gradual loss of active haemopoietic tissue initially in the long bones and later in the flat bones; vertebral marrow persists till death.
2 The cellular composition of the residual haemopoietic tissue is normal and responds satisfactorily to the usual stimuli such as erythropoietin, anoxia and blood loss.

Absorption of haematinics
1 Usually the essential haematinics can be absorbed without difficulty from an ordinary mixed 'European' diet.
2 Deficiencies occur when there is poverty, self-neglect, food faddism, alcoholism and mental or physical illness.
3 Atrophic gastritis, anatomical abnormalities such as duodenal or jejunal diverticula and previous surgery, especially gastrectomy, may lead to malabsorption.

Anaemia in the elderly

Normal old people are not anaemic and have haemoglobin levels compatible with the World Health Organization (WHO) recommended minimum levels of 13 g/dl for men and 12 g/dl for women, although there is some individual variation. Anaemia is prevalent and often multifactorial. Both the prevalence and the complexity of anaemia tend to increase with the age of the population studied. The incidence of anaemia in both community and hospital surveys varies enormously on account of the different methodologies and the populations studied. The main causes of anaemia are:

Excess red cell loss
1 Bleeding: recent acute or chronic.
2 Haemolysis: Uncommon in 'pure' form but may compound anaemia due to another cause, e.g. malignant disease, drugs, cold agglutinins.

Impaired red cell formation
1 Deficiency disorders: lack of iron, vitamin B_{12}, vitamin C, folic acid or protein.
2 Other causes of marrow dysfunction, secondary to chronic disease, marrow depression or invasion.
The morphological type will give clues to the aetiology (Table 17.1). There is considerable geographical variation in the incidence of the different types and combined forms are not uncommon.

Table 17.1. Morphology suggests aetiology

Normocytic and usually normochromic
1 Acute blood loss; likely to be obvious on other grounds.
2 Secondary anaemia, e.g. chronic infection, collagen disease, malignancy, protein malnutrition.

Microcytic and usually hypochromic
1 Chronic blood loss and/or inadequate iron intake.
2 Occasionally normochromic and secondary.

Macrocytic
1 Normoblastic, e.g. posthaemorrhagic, haemolytic, leukoerythroblastic; secondary to hypothyroidism, liver disease, scurvy and alcohol abuse.
2 Megaloblastic, e.g. pernicious anaemia, folate deficiency.

Investigation of anaemia
1 The routine clinical work-up usually reveals both the severity and the cause of the anaemia; ask especially about diet, drugs, alcohol and tobacco.
2 If iron deficiency is likely, seek evidence of previous gastric surgery, malignant disease and blood in the stool, but remember that bleeding may be intermittent.
3 More specialized investigations may be required to explore the results of the initial work-up.

Iron deficiency anaemia

Aetiology
1 Iron deficiency anaemia is usually due to chronic blood loss especially from the gastrointestinal tract and less often from the genito-urinary tract or elsewhere.

2 Defective absorption may be a contributory (rarely the sole) factor on account of chronic gastritis, gastrectomy or small bowel disease. Look for clinical or biochemical evidence of malabsorption such as steatorrhoea, osteomalacia and vitamin B deficiencies.
3 Inadequate intake may stem from inability to cope as a result of physical or mental disorder or from poverty.

Clinical picture
There may be complaints of the underlying disorder or simply non-specific ill health such as 'going off', weakness, falls or possibly congestive cardiac failure. The time-honoured hallmarks of chronic sideropenia are rarely seen.

Investigation
The peripheral blood picture will show hypochromia. It is not usually necessary to investigate iron status. Radiology and endoscopy may be indicated to diagnose the underlying disorder. Remember that a benign upper gastrointestinal lesion such as an hiatus hernia may conceal a more serious lesion lower down, e.g. carcinoma of the colon.

Treatment
1 Treat the cause.
2 Give oral iron to bring the haemoglobin up to normal and continue for at least another 3 months to replenish the body stores.
3 If the response is not satisfactory check that the patient is taking the tablets and that the diagnosis is correct. Consider the possibility of continued blood loss or other factors, which may have been overlooked, such as chronic infection, malignancy, renal disease or malabsorption.
4 If there is genuine intolerance to the oral iron or serious defect in patient compliance give parenteral iron as a total dose infusion or by repeated intramuscular injections. Follow the manufacturer's instructions meticulously.
5 Blood transfusion, using packed cells and a diuretic, may be necessary if there is need to correct the anaemia urgently.

Sideroblastic anaemia

Acquired sideroblastic anaemia is a disease of later life. It is due to impaired utilization rather than lack of iron. The sideroblasts in the marrow are erythroblasts containing excess iron. The primary form may masquerade as 'refractory' iron deficiency or even megaloblastic anaemia. The RBCs are predominantly normochromic but may be macrocytic and it is necessary to exclude coexisting folate and B_{12} deficiencies. The secondary form is seen in association with a variety of disorders including myeloproliferative disorder, malignancy, collagen disease and myxoedema.

Treatment is for the associated pathology but in addition pyridoxine, folic acid and repeated blood transfusions are employed. The latter should be kept to a minimum because of iron overload.

Anaemia of chronic disease

This is common in elderly patients and often coexists with other types of anaemia. The patient often experiences great lassitude. The peripheral blood picture may not give a clear indication of the likely cause, being hypochromic, normochromic, or occasionally macrocytic. The anaemia tends to be refractory because although there is sufficient iron available the reticuloendothelial system is unable adequately to utilize it. The serum ferritin levels are normal or raised and the TIBC is low in contrast to iron deficiency. It is often associated with protein calorie malnutrition, with hypoalbuminaemia and lymphocytopenia. Common examples are:

1 Rheumatoid arthritis
In addition to 'anaemia of chronic disease', look for blood loss (antirheumatic drugs), inadequate nutrition and for folate or B_{12} deficiency. Low folate may be due to reduced intake and increased utilization. Complications of rheumatoid disease such as vasculitis or amyloidosis increase the severity and complexity of the anaemia.

2 Malignant disease
Usually a combination of causes will be operative: anorexia, blood loss, 'anaemia of chronic disease', malabsorption and haemolysis. Additionally, there may be marrow infiltration with development of a leucoerythroblastic anaemia.

3 Renal disease
Anaemia increases with the severity of chronic renal failure and is usually normochromic and normocytic. Additional factors include

blood loss, haemolysis and marrow failure. The latter becomes dominant in the end stages. A normal haemoglobin suggests that the renal failure is acute and reversible. Some normoblastic anaemias respond more readily to treatment of the underlying disorder. For example:

(a) Hypothyroidism. The macrocytic normoblastic anaemia which occurs in over 50 per cent of cases in myxoedema is usually mild, never megaloblastic and responds slowly to thyroxine. Coexisting iron deficiency will require treatment. About 10 per cent of cases also have Addisonian pernicious anaemia (PA).

(b) Scurvy. The macrocytic normoblastic anaemia of scurvy is commonly associated with other nutritional deficiencies. Vitamin C replacement followed by a proper diet is curative.

Megaloblastic anaemia

The megaloblastic anaemias are due to deficiency of vitamin B_{12} or folic acid. They are much less common than anaemia due to iron deficiency or chronic disease.

Vitamin B_{12} deficiency

Addisonian pernicious anaemia (PA), incidence 1 per cent over age 60, is the usual cause of vitamin B_{12} deficiency but other causes are gastrectomy, bacterial colonization of intestinal strictures or diverticula and disorders of the terminal ileum. Vegans can use Cytacon oral liquid preparation prophylactically but not if they develop PA or other cause of malabsorption of B_{12}.

Pernicious anaemia

Pernicious anaemia develops insidiously due to auto-immune gastric atrophy and failure of intrinsic factor secretion. Cancer of the stomach is said to occur in 10 per cent of cases. Other complications are peripheral neuropathy, subacute combined degeneration of the spinal cord and mental disorder. Clinical features include:
- Symptoms and signs of anaemia with yellow tinge to skin.
- Glossitis, anorexia and weight loss.
- In severe cases hepatosplenomegaly, heart failure.

Diagnosis of PA
1 There is a macrocytic anaemia, a low serum B_{12} and a megaloblastic marrow.
2 The Dicopac double radio-isotope test will confirm that B_{12} can be absorbed only when given with intrinsic factor. The test is not necessary in most cases.
3 Antibodies to gastric parietal cells are found in the serum in 90 per cent, to intrinsic factor in 60 per cent and to thyroid in 40 per cent of cases.

Treatment of B_{12} deficiency
1 Hydroxocobalamin intramuscularly every 3–4 days initially to replenish body stores, thereafter every 3–4 months for life.
2 There is often associated iron deficiency necessitating oral iron.
3 Blood transfusion is generally not indicated.

Folate deficiency

Folate deficiency is much more common than B_{12} deficiency and is usually due to poor diet with or without malabsorption. Other factors are increased demand (lymphoma, neoplasm, infection, haemolysis), anticonvulsant drugs and chronic alcoholism. The clinical features include:
1 Irritability, depression, mental confusion and occasionally dementia.
2 Peripheral neuropathy and subacute combined degeneration of the cord (as with PA) in more severe cases.

Diagnosis
The peripheral blood-and-marrow picture is identical to that of B_{12} deficiency. Measurement of vitamin levels in the blood (no anti-biotics for at least 24 hours) allows the distinction to be made. The red cell folate is low. Folic acid absorption tests are not used routinely.

Treatment of folate deficiency
1 Correct the aberrant lifestyle—poor diet, alcohol abuse; stop offending drugs when practicable.
2 Oral folic acid tablets for a few months to replenish stores, then stop; long-term use may mask developing PA.

3 Do not give folate until B_{12} deficiency excluded—risk of precipitating subacute combined degeneration of the cord. If in doubt give both vitamins concurrently; may need iron also.

4 Use of folic acid is more hazardous than the other haematinics. May be justified prophylactically in malabsorption states and epileptics on anticonvulsants.

Marrow failure

Severe forms of marrow failure are rather rare but may occur from drug treatment or marrow replacement, e.g. myelofibrosis, leukaemia and secondary carcinoma. Moderate cases appear from time to time, and the mild forms in otherwise healthy old people have earned the sobriquet 'the anaemia of senescence'. The cause is not apparent in at least 50 per cent of cases but consider:

• Drugs such as sulphonamides both antibiotic and antidiabetic, anticonvulsants, phenothiazines, antirheumatics and of course, known cytotoxics. The aged marrow is particularly liable to be depressed by drugs.

• Unsuspected renal disease, low-grade myeloproliferative disorders and malignancies not invading the bones.

There is a pancytopenia in both the peripheral blood and the marrow and the low platelet and white cell counts put the patient at risk of bleeding and infection.

Treatment

1 Mild cases require no active treatment but remove all potential causative agents and any other medication unless strongly indicated.

2 Check B_{12}, folate and iron status or give standard haematinics because deficiency of one or more is so common.

3 Give prednisolone if a haemolytic element or auto-immune process is implicated.

4 Non-virilizing anabolic steroids or fluoxymesterone are often advocated.

5 Many cases appear to stabilize at the 8–10 g/dl level and may not require active treatment; otherwise give blood transfusions to bring the haemoglobin level up sufficiently to allow the patient to cope.

Leukaemia

All types of leukaemia have increased in incidence in the past 50–60 years, especially in the elderly who are most often affected by chronic lymphocytic and to a lesser extent acute myeloid leukaemia.

Acute leukaemia
1 Usually myeloblastic and may have an antecedent haematological disorder such as chronic myeloid leukaemia or primary polycythaemia.
2 The prognosis is poor with rapidly worsening anaemia, enlarged lymph nodes and thrombocytopenic purpura with spontaneous bleeding.
3 The leucocyte count is variable but there will be large numbers of primitive 'blast' cells. The platelet count is usually low and may lead to a prolonged bleeding time with poor clot retraction. The marrow picture is diagnostic.
4 Treatment is with general supportive measures; combination chemotherapy is arduous for all concerned.

Chronic lymphocytic leukaemia (CLL)
CLL increases in incidence with age and is the commonest of the lymphoproliferative disorders. B–cells usually predominate, hypogamma-globulinaemia is common and there is reduced immunocompetence. There may be an auto-immune haemolytic anaemia with a positive Coombs test. The WBC is usually very high and most cells are lymphocytes. The clinical picture includes:
• An insidious, benign course extending over very many years.
• Increasing normochromic anaemia, lymphadenopathy, splenomegaly with or without hepatomegaly.
• Liability to herpes zoster and recurrent infections.
• Death from an unrelated cause in the benign cases or from intercurrent infection, leukaemic infiltration, thrombocytopenic purpura or haemolytic crisis.

Treatment of CLL
1 No treatment needed if disease not progressive.
2 Chlorambucil or cyclophosphamide if disease produces symptoms.

3 Steroids for haemolytic anaemia and thrombocytopenia.
4 Antibiotics for intercurrent infections.

Chronic myeloid leukaemia (CML)

CML also affects especially the elderly but is not so common as CLL and the mean survival time is much less. An acute myeloblastic phase is a common terminal event. The WBC is very high, mostly segmented neutrophils. The clinical features include:

- Weakness, haemorrhage, infection.
- Moderate lymphadenopathy and gross splenomegaly.
- Evidence of leukaemic deposits in skin, brain or bone.

Atypical cases cause difficulty and tend to occur in the elderly. There may be little or no hepatosplenomegaly, a much lower WBC count, features of myelofibrosis or polycythaemia (see below) and a raised leucocyte alkaline phosphatase count (it is typically low in CML). Treatment is usually with busulphan; most patients have a worthwhile response. Hyperuricaemia should be corrected before the cytotoxic is given and during treatment, using allopurinol. Infection is less of a problem than with CLL. Removal or irradiation of the spleen is occasionally indicated.

Raised haemoglobin

Relative erythrocytosis is mostly due to dehydration and intravascular volume depletion. This may occur in the old person who has no thirst and lives with persistent hydropenia which is rapidly exacerbated by illness. Such patients have an increased risk of stroke. Rehydration can be achieved and maintained only by encouragement.

Secondary erythrocytosis is a physiological response to chronic anoxaemia and high levels of erythropoietin. Treatment is that of the underlying disorder.

Primary polycythaemia

A rather rare myeloproliferative disorder with a maximum incidence age 50 to 80 years. There is an increased cell mass affecting red and white cells and platelets. It occasionally progresses to chronic myeloid leukaemia or myelofibrosis. Definitive investigation is by measurement of the red cell mass as a proportion of lean body mass. The clinical picture is due to the increased blood volume, hyperviscosity, engorgement of vessels and tissue hypoxia, viz:

- Hypertension with liability to thromboses (e.g. stroke, myocardial infarct) or haemorrhage especially from gastrointestinal or renal tracts.
- Florid, cynanosed facies, pruritus, splenomegaly, low ESR.

Treatment apart from repeated venesection to give rapid, temporary relief, requires specialist involvement, may include:

1 IV radioactive phosphorus.
2 Chemotherapy with busulphan or chlorambucil.
3 Iron, anticoagulants, allopurinol to prevent gout, and cholestyramine for pruritus.

Multiple myeloma

Myelomatosis is a malignant proliferation of a single clone (occasionally two clones) of plasma cell precursors (myeloma cells) which produce abnormal proteins (paraproteins). It is more common than CLL and has the highest incidence in the over 70s. For information on paraproteinaemia refer to standard texts. There is a long pre-clinical phase which may last for many years, with the diagnosis being made fortuitously. In the clinical phase there is increasing ill health with:

- Anaemia, bone pain, pathological fracture, especially ribs, femur and vertebrae.
- Nausea, vomiting and mental disturbance due to renal failure or hypercalcaemia.
- Immune paresis with infections.
- Progressive renal failure from the effects of paraproteins, hypercalcaemia and amyloidosis.
- Peripheral neuropathy, paraplegia from spinal deposits and vertebral collapse.

The diagnosis is confirmed by examination of the marrow but may already be evident from the very high ESR, raised globulins with monoclonal band on electrophoresis and possibly skeletal lesions on X-ray. Bence–Jones proteinuria (light kappa or lambda chains), present in about 50 per cent of cases, is virtually diagnostic. Life expectancy from time of diagnosis is less than 2 years and increasing uraemia indicates a grave prognosis. Treatment may require specialist help:

1 No specific treatment usually in the pre-clinical phase; maintain

high fluid intake to prevent hypercalcaemia and renal failure.

2 Melphalan to damp down the plasmacytosis.

3 Prednisolone to reduce hypercalcaemia and enhance response to melphalan.

4 NSAIDs, opiates and local irradiation for bone pain.

5 Allopurinol to control hyperuricaemia, blood transfusion for anaemia and antibiotics for intercurrent infections.

6 Plasmapheresis for hyperviscosity.

Further reading

Hyams D.E. (1985) The Blood. In: Brocklehurst J.C. (ed.) *Textbook of Geriatric Medicine and Gerontology*, pp. 835–98. Churchill Livingstone, Edinburgh.

Lipschitz D.A. (1985) Anaemia. In: Exton-Smith A.N. & Weksler M.E. (eds) *Practical Geriatric Medicine*, pp. 290–6. Churchill Livingstone, Edinburgh.

Chapter 18
Cancer (Malignant Disease)

About half of all cancer in the Western world occurs in those aged 65 years or older. In the UK population of this age, cancer is the second main cause of death after cardiovascular disease; in younger women over the age of 30 it is the prime cause. After age 65 the incidence of cancer in men increasingly outstrips that in women. The age-specific incidence and mortality for all the major malignancies increase with age except for acute lymphatic leukaemia, Hodgkin's disease, primary bone and joint tumours and testicular cancer, see Fig. 18.1.

About 60 per cent of all cancer mortality in Britain is attributable to 4 sites: the lung, breast, stomach and colo-rectum. These cancers are all frequently encountered in old people. Other common sites in this age group are skin, prostate, uterus and bladder. Hypotheses to explain the increased incidence of cancer with age include:

1 Long life gives longer exposure to carcinogenic influences such as background radiation, actinic light, diet and cigarette smoke.
2 Failing immunological surveillance.
3 Changes in hormonal balance.

There is debate as to whether cancer is generally more, or less aggressive in the older patient. Unfortunately there are no adequate data based on 'doubling time' studies to clarify this issue. Most clinical trials use the '5-year cure' as a yardstick which is not well suited to the very old. Malignant melanoma and thyroid cancer both appear to be more aggressive in the old than in the young, on the other hand carcinoma of the breast is more likely to be oestrogen receptor positive in the post-menopause and so have a better response to treatment.

Diagnosis

Early cancers may be discovered during the course of medical examination for some other reason, others are picked up on routine

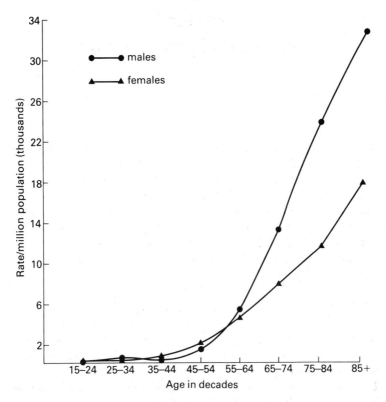

Fig. 18.1. Age-specific death rates for malignant disease. England 1985 (OPCS data).

screening or 'health checks' but many present too late for curative therapy. Delay in diagnosis may be due to:

1 Fear of knowing the diagnosis; victim likely to know people of own age who have died from cancer and so does not consult doctor.

2 Non-specific presentation with common symptoms, e.g. mental confusion, feeling 'off colour', poor appetite, weight loss or concern about the bowels. There are many possible causes for these.

3 The symptoms (even the signs) may be submerged in a sea of multiple pathology.

4 The doctor who does not recognize the significance of the symptoms and signs, or who fails to take early appropriate action. This is hardly surprising having regard to 2 and 3 above. The GP will see innumerable patients with mental confusion, 'bad stomach',

'bad chest' or 'trouble with the bowels' before encountering gastric, bronchogenic or colo-rectal cancer.

Even with a high level of suspicion concerning an underlying malignancy, it can be problematical as to how aggressively to pursue the diagnosis. Fortunately with modern technology both the nature and extent of the disease often can be assessed without great stress to the patient. This information is invaluable for appropriate treatment, prognosis and in the advice to be given to patient and relatives. The patient's affairs may be handled quite differently if it is known that the collapsed vertebral bodies are due to malignancy rather than to osteoporosis.

Treatment

General considerations

● Quality rather than quantity of life is of paramount importance in this age group.

● A supportive team approach is required to provide counselling to patients, relatives and friends and to cover all aspects of care.

● Surgical extirpation of the lesion is rarely precluded on grounds of age alone. With meticulous pre- and post-operative treatment the acute stress of the operation may be better tolerated than the more prolonged stress of radiotherapy or cytotoxic drug therapy.

● Radiotherapy and chemotherapy have the same effects on the various cancers as in the young but the effect on the patient's normal tissues is enhanced and patients who appear 'aged' in biological terms suffer more from adverse effects. Modification of the treatment is required and this may impair the curative effects. The balance has to be struck with care.

● Palliative radiotherapy can be highly satisfactory for the relief of local pressure effects, obstruction and pain.

● A major problem is marrow suppression and allowance must always be made in chemotherapy for the age-related reduction of renal function which will be present even in those without evidence of renal disease.

● Adverse effects which may be acceptable in a young person with ample physiological reserves could prove to be a disaster for an old person just capable of self-care. Even a moderate amount of peripheral neuropathy induced by vincristine could knock an elderly person off her feet if she already has poor balance and weak muscles. Most chemocurable malignancies occur in younger patients. Cytotoxic chemotherapy in the elderly is focused on lympho-myeloproliferative disorders but is also used for palliation, e.g. in carcinoma of breast, lung (small cell) and ovary.

• The presence of associated diseases must be taken into account when planning treatment because of the extra liability to adverse effects; for example patients with impaired cardiac, respiratory or renal function.

• Polypharmacy poses hazards with chemotherapeutic agents, for example:

(i) Aspirin and NSAIDs can increase methotrexate toxicity.

(ii) Allopurinol can increase toxicity of cyclophosphamide and 6–mercaptopurine.

(iii) Oral hypoglycaemic drugs can be potentiated by cyclophosphamide.

Reactions to radiation and chemotherapy

In addition to the non-specific acute inflammatory reactions with radiotherapy the major effects are on actively dividing cells especially skin, bone marrow, gastrointestinal tract and gonads. The adverse effects can be severe with curative doses but are seldom such a problem with palliative treatment. General systemic effects are fatigue, anorexia, nausea and vomiting and mental depression. The latter may be relieved by allowing the patient to 'talk through' her problems and also by the use of antidepressants. Nausea and vomiting are treated with the centrally acting phenothiazines, metoclopramide (which also has a peripheral action on the gut), domperidone (less central effects) or the cannabinoid nabilone.

Oncological emergencies

The management of cancer is a relatively long-term affair but on occasion swift action is essential to prevent unnecessary loss of mental or physical function and to avert premature death with:

• Infection.
• Hypercalcaemia.
• Electrolyte imbalance.
• Spinal cord compression.
• Superior mediastinal and vena caval obstruction.
• Pathological fracture.

In addition concomitant medical emergencies may require treatment. A balanced approach is essential to improve the quality of life remaining. Is the treatment likely to provide comfort as well as preservation of function or will it just prolong the misery of dying? These humane, ethical questions must not be overlooked. Symptom control is the supreme good in disseminated cancer.

Some common cancers

Figure 18.2 illustrates the incidence of the most common cancers in East Anglia. Apart from carcinoma of the cervix they are all more common in the elderly. Cancers of the lung, trachea and bronchus and cancers of the skin top the list. For these cancers, males predominate (except for malignant melanoma) but female rates are increasing faster. Thus in the past 25 years in this region, the female

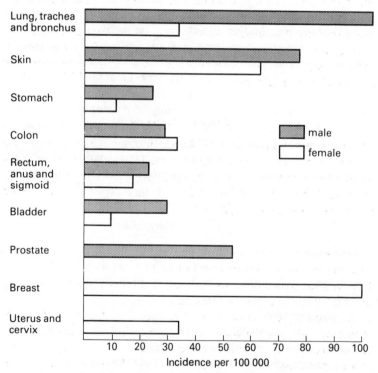

Fig. 18.2. Common cancers in East Anglia (1985).

rates for lung cancer have trebled, those for basal cell carcinoma and squamous cell carcinoma have more than doubled and for malignant melanoma have more than quadrupled. By contrast the rates for males appear to have stabilized for lung and to be increasing less quickly for skin cancers.

Bronchogenic cancer

The major cancer of old age in men, mostly due to tobacco smoking but occasionally due to industrial exposure to asbestos, arsenic, nickel, chromates and other substances.

Diagnosis and treatment
Diagnosis is usually straightforward using X-ray, sputum cytology and bronchoscopy, but unless surgical removal is practicable it may not be worthwhile submitting the patient to endoscopy. Not only must the tumour be resectable and without metastases but there needs to be sufficient remaining lung function. Ultrasound, CT and bone scan may be used to delineate the full extent of the disease. The general prognosis is poor and even worse for the small cell variety. Radiotherapy can give relief to both obstructive symptoms and pain from metastases.

Cancer of the breast

The most common cancer of women in later life. The prognosis relates to the extent of the disease, especially axillary node involvement, when first seen. Some patients live for many years without treatment but the median survival time after recurrence or metastases is less than 2 years.

Management
Primary carcinoma of breast
1 Diagnosis, often obvious but may be confirmed histologically by needle biopsy or at time of ablation.
2 Tamoxifen (see below) is the first line of treatment for the more elderly or others for whom surgery and radiotherapy is unsuitable; about 60 per cent respond to some degree.
3 'Lumpectomy' and radiotherapy may be employed for the younger, fitter patients.

Recurrent carcinoma of the breast

1 Tamoxifen again is the first choice for the post-menopausal woman and about 30 per cent will respond.

2 Relapse of an initially sensitive tumour may be controlled for a time by the expert oncologist 'ringing the changes' on other hormonal and chemotherapeutic agents.

3 Radiotherapy can be used to treat pain from bony metastases, to forestall ulceration or to shrink a tumour which has ulcerated.

4 Aminoglutethimide produces a medical 'adrenalectomy' and also inhibits the conversion of androgens to oestrogens in the peripheral tissues; corticosteroid replacement therapy is required.

Tamoxifen is an antioestrogen which may also have cytocidal effects. It has a long half-life and a steady state is not reached for at least 6 weeks after the start of treatment. The clinical response is to be expected over a period of months rather than weeks. It is widely used because of its efficacy and minimal toxicity. Most post-menopausal women take it without much upset. However there may be worsening temporarily of pain from the malignant lesions as well as hypercalcaemia and fluid retention.

Cancer of the female genital tract

Bleeding from the genital tract long after the menopause must always be taken seriously because there may be pre-malignant or malignant disease as well as benign causes. The patient will present stained underwear or bed sheets, but if she is also incontinent of urine or has an anal lesion the source of the loss may not be immediately obvious; however the history and physical examination should make this clear. The heavier the bleeding the more likely the cause is malignant.

Ask especially about hormone-replacement therapy which is increasingly common, also trauma. Even very old ladies can be subject to the latter either from coitus after a long period of abstinence or from some foreign body in the vagina, the commonest being a long-forgotten ring pessary. Further investigation is the province of the gynaecologist and likely causes for bleeding are:

• Atrophic vaginitis which will respond to topical oestrogen cream.

• Benign tumours such as cervical or endometrial polyps.

• Endometrial hyperplasia which may be pre-malignant.

• Cancer of the genital tract involving vulva, vagina, cervix or endometrium.

Cancer of the prostate

This disease is the third most common cause of death from cancer in men over the age of 55 years, and is exceedingly common in those over 70 years with an incidence of latent cancer in clinical series of 20–40 per cent (see Fig. 18.3). Patients usually present with prostatism (see Chapter 16) or bone pain from metastases and over 50 per cent have spread beyond the prostate when first seen. With invasive disease the median duration of first remission is no more than 1 to 2 years and the mean survival time is about 4 years. The diagnosis is based on palpation of the gland, ultrasonography using a rectal probe and histology from needle biopsy or transurethral resection (TUR) of the obstruction. Bony metastases may be recognized on the skeletal X–ray but the bone scan is much more sensitive. CT will detect metastases in pelvic and para-aortic nodes.

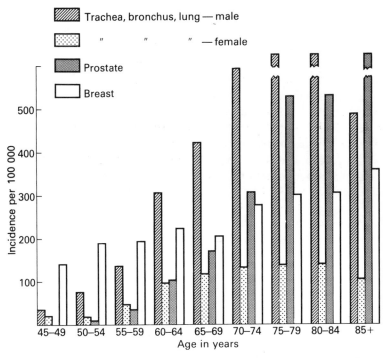

Fig. 18.3. Age-specific (incidence) rate of three common cancers in East Anglia (1985).

Treatment
1 Treatment can relieve symptoms but does little to prolong survival.
2 No treatment is given if the patient is asymptomatic and there is no spread outside of the prostate.
3 TUR is necessary to relieve bladder-neck obstruction.
4 If there is evidence of spread beyond the gland, hormone therapy generally is indicated, but not all would agree with treatment in the absence of symptoms even at this stage.
5 Radical prostatectomy gives no better results and the morbidity is greater than with hormonal manipulation.
6 Radiotherapy is also used, especially for the anaplastic tumour (even when still confined to the prostate) and for localized metastases.
7 Occasional blood transfusions are helpful for the patient with slowly progressive metastatic disease and severe anaemia.

Hormonal manipulation
The aim is to reduce the androgen stimulation of the tumour; hormonal manipulations include:

First-line treatment
- Bilateral subcapsular orchidectomy.
- Diethylstilboestrol but risk of thromboembolism.

Second-line treatment
- Cyproterone acetate, an antiandrogen.
- Longacting gonadotrophin-releasing hormone analogues, via injection or snuff; these are very expensive and not generally available.
- Aminoglutethimide which inhibits adrenal steroid production (medical adrenalectomy) and corticosteroid replacement will be required.

Gastrointestinal cancers

See also Chapter 14.

Oesophageal cancer
Usually a squamous cell, less often adenocarcinoma and is about

twice as common in men. The main aetiological factors are:
- Chronic oesophagitis including excessive use of tobacco and alcohol.
- Nitrosamines in food.
- Longstanding sideropenia.

The clinical presentation includes dysphagia for solids, weight loss, chest pain and aspiration pneumonia. Some lesions are operable, others are best treated conservatively. Radiotherapy is helpful for the squamous type. If the lumen is narrowed to a critical degree the insertion of a plastic (Celestin) tube is advisable and especially prior to radiotherapy which might cause swelling of the growth and totally block the gullet. Never advise gastrostomy!

Gastric carcinoma
Reducing in incidence but is still quite common; the rate for men is about twice that for women. The peak incidence is in the eighth decade. There is a genetic predisposition, an association with blood group A and atrophic gastritis, and also considerable geographical variation in incidence. Clinically indigestion, weight loss, vomiting, haematemesis and melaena, and abdominal pain may occur. The diagnosis is confirmed by endoscopy or barium meal, the prognosis is poor and the treatment usually palliative and may include gastrectomy.

Carcinoma of the colon and rectum
An adenocarcinoma with a relatively low grade of malignancy. Patients with Crohn's disease and more especially those with polyposis and chronic ulcerative colitis are at increased risk of developing colo-rectal cancer.

The clinical presentation is often rather vague but malaise, abdominal pain and change of bowel habit, rectal bleeding, tenesmus or faecal incontinence, depending on the site of the lesion, are the usual pointers. The diagnosis is confirmed by sigmoidoscopy and barium enema or colonoscopy. We regard the two latter investigations as inpatient procedures for the very old, partly to ensure adequate bowel preparation and also to reduce the stress on the patient. Treatment is surgical resection.

Malignant diseases of the skin
The predisposing factor is excessive exposure to actinic light.

Present-day wanton exposure to the sun must surely produce a massive increase in the incidence of these malignancies. Caucasian people in tropical and subtropical climates enjoying the outdoor life are at maximum risk. Even in the UK there is a demonstrable increase in incidence from north to south (see also Chapter 19).

Basal cell carcinoma (BCC)

The most common and readily recognizable as a pearly papule which slowly but relentlessly grows and develops a central area of necrosis (the rodent ulcer). The usual site is the upper face, often in a slightly shaded area such as the inner canthus. Metastases are rare but local invasion can cause great destruction. Early curettage and cautery is the treatment of choice but very thin lesions respond to fluorouracil cream. The prognosis is good; late lesions require surgery or radiotherapy.

Squamous cell carcinoma (Scc)

Arises especially from damaged skin, e.g. leukoplakia or solar keratosis (eradicable at the pre-malignant stage with fluorouracil cream) on sites exposed to maximum sunshine such as the head, pinnae, neck, backs of hands and lips. It grows more rapidly than BCC and is liable to metastasize to regional lymph nodes, especially from the ear. The initial appearance is a reddened induration. Early surgery plus radiotherapy gives a good prognosis.

Malignant melanoma

A more rare and difficult tumour to recognize. It has a much worse prognosis than BCC or SCC. Many common benign skin lesions in the elderly are pigmented, e.g. moles, naevi, thrombosed warts and seborrhoeic keratosis; when in doubt refer to the dermatologist. Definitive treatment is wide excision and skin graft. Metastases commonly occur but radiotherapy and chemotherapy are not generally of much help.

Further reading

Brada M. & Horwich A. (1986) Oncological emergencies. *Hospital Update*, **12**, 799–812.

Cohen H.J. & Crawford J. (1985) Cancer. In: Exton-Smith A.N. & Weskler M.E. (eds) *Practical Geriatric Medicine*, pp. 57–65. Churchill Livingstone, Edinburgh.

Consumers' Association (1986) Management of metastatic prostatic carcinoma. *Drug and Therapeutics Bulletin*, **224**, 85–7.

Consumers' Association (1986) Tamoxifen in breast cancer. *Drug and Therapeutics Bulletin*, **24**, 65–7.

Rees J.G. (1987) What chemotherapy can do for elderly patients. *Geriatric Medicine*, **17**, 70–6.

Chapter 19
Eyes, Ears, Mouth and Skin

Eyes

Age changes

1 Eyes appear sunken in old age due to loss of peri-orbital fat.
2 Arcus senilis is common but not significant.
3 The pupils tend to be small and slow to react to light and accommodation becomes impaired. Dilatation is also poor and hinders adaptation to dark.
4 The lens becomes inelastic; focusing, especially on near objects becomes difficult.
5 Entropion (inturned lashes) is common and causes irritation of the cornea.
6 Ectropion (out-turned lashes) is common and the most frequent cause of epiphora (watery eye).

Examination of the retinal fundus in old age
Shortacting eye drops are recommended, e.g. topicamide 0.5 per cent. Reversal with pilocarpine is usually unnecessary and can be painful. The risk of acute closed angle ('congestive') glaucoma is minimal, but beware the small eyeball with a shallow anterior chamber and small diameter cornea. If in doubt, dilate only one pupil with phenylephrine 10 per cent and reverse with thymoxamine 0.5 per cent and leave the other eye for a subsequent occasion.

Loss of vision
Approximately 70000 persons over the age of 65 years in the UK are registered as partially sighted, i.e. about 1 per cent of the elderly population. Many more are visually disabled but remain unregistered. Registration of disability is an essential qualification for special supplementary benefits and aids.

Visual impairment

Slow loss	*Sudden loss*
Open angle glaucoma (chronic)	Arterial occlusion
Cataracts	Venous occlusion
Macular degeneration	Retinal detachment
Iatrogenic disease	Haemorrhage
Retinopathy (DM)	Acute glaucoma

NB   If one eye is affected the other is at risk.

The painful eye
1 Closed angle glaucoma (acute).
2 Infection:
  Conjunctivitis
  Uveitis
  Herpes zoster.
3 Trauma—foreign body.

Glaucoma
See Table 19.1.

Table 19.1. Glaucoma

	Acute—closed angle	Chronic—open angle
Symptoms	Sudden pain in eye, blurred vision, vomiting and prostration	Insidious loss of vision leading to tunnel vision
Signs	Eye tense, irregular fixed pupil, cornea and conjunctivae congested	Raised pressure on tonometry, scotoma on field testing
Pathology	Sudden impairment of anterior chamber drainage—may be precipitated by anticholingerics and mydriatrics	Gradual increase in intraocular pressure—idiopathic
Treatment	Constricted pupil, analgesia, diuretics	Pilocarpine drops, drainage operation

Cataracts

Types
(i) Central—early visual loss.

(ii) Peripheral—late visual loss and vision impaired by scattering of bright light.

Causes
?Ageing.
Hereditary.
Diabetes mellitus.
Iatrogenic, e.g. steroids.

Treatment
Central type—dilatation of pupil improves vision, e.g. homatro-pine.
Peripheral—avoid bright glaring light.

Surgery
Only needed when patient is handicapped and quality of life is impaired.

Contraindications
(i) Early stages.
(ii) Where macular degeneration is known also to be present.
(iii) In the presence of severe mental impairment.

Surgical procedures
Removal of cataract plus provision of aphakic glasses or
Provision of contact lenses or
Implantation of artificial lens—first choice where good facilities are available.

Complications of treatment
(i) Dilatation of pupil—may precipitate glaucoma.
(ii) Aphakic glasses—leads to visual distortion and restriction of visual fields.
(iii) Contact lenses—good dexterity needed and perseverance if successful use is to be achieved.
(iv) Lens implant—difficult, possible failure and risk of infection.

Treatable precipitating/aggravating factors in vascular causes of visual loss
1 Hypertension/hypotension.
2 Diabetes.

3 Polycythaemia.
4 Paraproteinaemia.
5 Arteritis.

Simple measures to assist patients with visual impairment
1 Check visual acuity—provision or change of lenses may help.
2 Keep patient and spectacles together.
3 Keep spectacles clean.
4 Insist on appropriate lighting—bright for some, avoid glare in others.
5 Register as partially sighted if sufficient impairment.
6 Seek low visual aid advice.
7 Maintain maximum hearing ability.
8 Seek support of blind association.
9 Subscribe to talking newspaper, talking book library, etc.

Ears

Ageing changes
1 Wax becomes more viscous.
2 Presbycusis occurs—loss of high frequency hearing.
3 Recruitment occurs, i.e. difficulty in hearing when background noise exists.

Deafness in old age
1 Deafness becomes more common with increasing age.
2 On formal testing just over half of geriatric patients have hearing impairment.
3 Of these with impairment one-half appear to cope well and feel that they have no need of help.
4 About one-quarter of geriatric patients would benefit and accept the provision of a hearing aid.

Causes of deafness

1 Nerve deafness
   Ageing (presbycusis)
   Ototoxicity—drugs, e.g. gentamycin and frusemide in high dosage
   Nerve compression, e.g. acoustic neuroma and Paget's disease

2 Conduction deafness

Otosclerosis—hereditary condition therefore early onset likely

Paget's disease of bone

Post-infective

At present only conductive forms of deafness are amenable to surgical treatment.

Management of deafness

1 Check for wax in ears—remove if present.

2 If deafness persists after wax removal—refer for audiometry.

3 If hearing aid provided—counsel about problems (i.e. an aid does not restore normal hearing).

4 Teach maintenance of aid, i.e. cleaning of tubing and battery replacement.

5 Follow up to ensure that aid is being used—volunteers can help.

6 Inform about environmental aids, e.g. flashing telephones and other adaptations, vibrating pillow alarm clock, loop system for TV, etc.

How to communicate with the deaf

1 Do not shout.

2 Speak clearly and slowly but not in an exaggerated way.

3 Do not sit with your back to the light, have your face well lit in order to assist lip reading.

4 Do not obscure or conceal your mouth, to do so makes lip reading difficult.

5 Ask the patient if she can hear you, adjust tone of voice, etc. if problem exists.

6 Check that if patient has an aid it is properly worn and functioning.

7 All clinics, consultation rooms and wards, should have available a simple portable microphone and ear piece.

8 If all else fails write down your questions.

Complications of deafness

1 Social isolation.

2 Psychiatric disorders, especially paranoia.

3 Associated tinnitus.

4 Associated dizziness and unsteadiness.

5 Increased risk of accidents because of reduced auditory warnings.

The mouth and its contents

1 Mucus membrane as site of disease
(i) Pemphygoid and pemphigus—blisters.
(ii) Lichen planus—white patches/ulceration.
(iii) Candida—white patches.
(iv) Aphthous ulcers—as in younger patients.

2 The tongue
(i) Smooth and shiny—iron deficiency.
(ii) Red and sore—glossitis, e.g. B–group deficiency.
(iii) Geographical/furred tongue—usually of no significance.
(iv) Fasciculation—motor neurone disease.
(v) Injury—think of epilepsy.
(vi) Ulceration—think of malignant disease.

3 The lips
(i) Herpes simplex—as in younger patients—often an indicator of systemic disease.
(ii) Angular stomatitis—usually due to escape of saliva due to poor closure— becomes red and sore, especially if complicated by fungal (candida) infection; most common in the edentulous.

4 The teeth
(i) Generally absent—95 per cent of geriatric patients are edentulous.
(ii) Any surviving teeth and the gums are usually in very poor condition, but attempts should always be made to preserve surviving teeth.
(iii) Sixty per cent of patients are unhappy with their dentures usually complaining of looseness.
(iv) Twelve per cent with dentures never wear them.
(v) The edentulous need to continue to consult dentists—gum ridges recede with age and new dentures will be needed.
(vi) Dentures should only be supplied to those who are prepared to wear them.
(vii) Dentures should always be removed when an airway is being maintained.
(viii) Dignity and nutrition are best maintained if well-fitting dentures are worn by the edentulous; the presence of surviving teeth help to secure a dental plate and improve the fit.

(ix) Dentures should be labelled to avoid loss if owner is admitted to an institution.

NB   In 'the wild'—non-accidental death (i.e. due to 'old age') is most commonly due to starvation secondary to dental loss.

The skin

Age changes

Confined to the dermis which becomes thinner, more transparent, more fragile and less elastic. The skin in old age is also drier and less greasy due to reduction in sebaceous excretion. Age related blemishes—of no significance are, e.g. senile purpura (on hands and forearms) Campbell de Morgan spots (on the trunk) sebaceous warts (face and back), telangiectasia (face).

Most age changes in the skin are proportional to the extent of environmental damage from sun and wind—or heat as in erythema ab igne.

Damage to skin

Leg ulcers and pressure sores are common, serious and expensive conditions in geriatric practice.

Leg ulcers

These are usually situated in the distal third of the lower leg. When associated with varicose veins, eczema and swollen ankles they are usually secondary to venous insufficiency. When well demarcated and painful, arterial insufficiency is most likely to be responsible. In many cases there will be a contribution from both venous and arterial disease.

Venous insufficiency	*Arterial insufficiency*
1 Associated ankle swelling.	1 Absent arterial pulses.
2 Associated varicose veins and varicose eczema.	2 In conditions with arteritis, e.g. rheumatoid arthritis.
3 Usually painless.	3 Often painful—especially in warmth and leg elevated.

Principles of treatment

1 Cleanse—saline, water or 1:20 Milton.
2 Apply—vaseline gauze or non-adherent dressing.

3 Cover—with gauze or gangee tissue.

4 Bandage—from toes to knee.

(i) Crepe bandage in presence of ischaemia or cellulitis.

(ii) Elastocrepe—in other instances.

5 Encourage mobility—but at rest elevate foot in venous ulcers.

6 Use antibiotics—after swab culture if cellulitis or toxicity are problems but beware of topical preparations because of risk of contact dermatitis.

7 Dressings should rarely be changed more frequently than once daily—when healing has started increase intervals between dressing changes.

Pressure sores

Areas of necrosis due to persistent and unrelieved pressure which exceeds the perfusion pressure of the tissues. The affected areas are usually between bony prominences and an unyielding surface upon which the patient is lying. Persistent moisture (e.g. incontinence) sheering forces (between the patient's skin and the supporting surface) are additional aggravating factors. In debilitated patients pressure sores may occur within hours but may take months to heal—or even prove fatal. Prevention is clearly cheaper and more humane than expensive and prolonged treatment. However, in many instances the damage may have occurred before presentation, e.g. during a 'long lie' after a fall at home. If prevention fails the extent of the damage must be restricted and healing then encouraged.

Preventive measures

1 Avoid falls, if possible.

2 Avoid immobility—in bed or chair.

Table 19.2. Method of scoring for vulnerability of developing pressure sores

Score	General physical condition	Mental state	Activity	Mobility	Incontinence
4	Good	Alert	Ambulant	Full	Not
3	Fair	Apathetic	Walks with help	Slightly limited	Occasionally
2	Poor	Confused	Chairbound	Very limited	Usually urine
1	Very bad	Stupor	Bedbound	Immobile	Doubly

Max. score 20, score of 14 or less indicates severe risk (after Exton–Smith, Norton & McLaren).

3 Relieve pressure—when immobility is unavoidable, e.g. by regular turning, mechanical devices (ripple mattress, water bed, suspension techniques) or protect vulnerable area, e.g. with foam or sheepskin.

4 Identify and protect at risk patients (Norton Scale)—see Table 19.2.

Limitation of damage

1 Maintain best possible perfusion pressure, i.e. support blood pressure and maintain good hydration.

2 Maintain good nutrition and maximum haemoglobin level, transfusing the patient, if necessary.

3 Keep area dry—catheterize, if necessary.

Encourage healing

1 Clean the sore, e.g. surgically by debridement or chemically with preparations, such as Eusol.

2 Use appropriate systemic antibiotics if there is an area of cellulitis or evidence of septicaemia; include treatment for anaerobic organisms.

3 Give nutritional supplements, including vitamin C and zinc.

4 Do not allow deep sores to become sealed off.

5 If the sore is large, clean and superficial grafting may be the quickest form of treatment.

Other important skin conditions in geriatric medicine

1 Shingles—the subsequent pain and debility present the most serious aspects of this condition. Treatment with antiviral preparations or steroids if started early (within 48 hours of onset of rash) may prevent or reduce the post-acute problems (see Chapter 11).

2 Pemphigus—this is a life-threatening condition which demands treatment with steroids. Pemphigoid is a similar but less severe condition.

3 Intertrigo—moist seborrhoeic eczema which is often secondarily infected with fungi. Improved personal hygiene and treatment with antifungal preparations will be required.

4 Basal cell carcinoma—especially where skin has been exposed to sunlight for prolonged and excessive periods for geographical or occupational reasons. See Chapter 18 for details of skin cancer.

5 Pruritus—search for systemic causes and infestations, also sensitivity reactions. Unfortunately many cases remain unexplained (senile pruritus).

6 Drug reactions—from eruptions to purpura. Pathological thinning of the skin secondary to steroid treatment is another common example.

7 Ulceration—secondary to trauma complicating other pathology.

Hair and nails

Age changes

Hair—becomes thinner, more brittle and loses its natural colour. Baldness may occur in both sexes but with differing distribution. Body hair is lost in the same order as its acquisition. Facial hair increases in women.

Nails—become thicker and harder—onychogryphosis when extreme.

Pathological changes
1 Retention of hair colour is said to indicate hypothyroidism.
2 Exaggerated hair loss may indicate hypopituitarism or be a consequence of cytotoxic therapy.
3 Toe nails may be neglected because of difficulty with maintenance due to visual impairment, arthritis or stroke disease.
4 Brittle and deformed nails may indicate systemic disease, e.g. deficiencies such as calcium or iron. Clubbing, pitting and white bands may indicate disease elsewhere.
5 Discomfort due to toe nail deformity and neglect can seriously impair mobility.
6 Extra care is needed in nail maintenance, in patients with peripheral vascular disease and neuropathy, e.g. diabetics.

Further reading

Monk B. & Brincat M. (1983) Ageing and the skin. *British J. Hospital Medicine,* **March.**

Solomon G. (1986) Hearing problems and the elderly. *Danish Medical Bulletin,* Gerontology Special Supplement series, **3.**

Chapter 20
Medical and Surgical Treatment
of the Old

Old people are not a homogeneous group. As age increases biological and social parameters of significance in clinical management become more disparate. Attention has already been drawn to the clinically relevant age changes and to the more common diseases which afflict the old.

A balanced approach to medical and surgical treatment

Age alone is virtually never a bar to medical or surgical treatment, nor should social circumstances or psychopathology blur our appreciation of the key medical issues. The balanced approach for the clinician is to:
- Make the correct diagnosis.
- Decide what medicine or surgery has to offer, curatively or palliatively.
- Consider to what extent the effects of age, psychosocial circumstances or other factors should modify the medical or surgical treatment plan.

This logical progression, focusing on the individual patient's needs should be incorporated into every clinical discussion and decision. Because of the multifactorial nature of the task good teamwork is essential whether in general practice or in hospital. Ideally the patient and the most concerned carers should also be involved in the discussions, which are too important to be left solely to doctors and other care practitioners. It is crucial to remember that very few old people want to die when feeling reasonably well. Relief from pain or from the toxicity of infection can transform attitudes to survival.

The case conference
The hospital or family practice team should hold regular case conferences with the purpose of achieving a balanced approach, to

217

probe the way forward, to implement decisions and to ensure that each member of the team knows what is going on and why. Answers are required to many questions such as: What happens next? How long before the patient returns to independence? What are the attitudes of the key supporters? And so on. It is crucial to answer

Table 20.1. Geriatric pharmacology

Age changes	Clinical effects
Pharmacokinetics	
Absorption from gut	
Passive transfer ⟷	Most drugs ⟷*
Active transfer ↓	Iron, calcium, thiamine, glucose ↓
Body composition	
Total body mass ↓	Blood drug levels generally ↑
Lean body mass ↓	Volume of distribution of lipid
Body fat ↑	soluble drugs ↑
Plasma albumin ↓	Plasma protein binding ↓ e.g. some
	sulphas, warfarin
Liver metabolism	First pass clearance ↓ e.g. oral
Oxidation ↓	anticoagulants, antidiabetics,
	propranolol and many psychotropics
Hydrolysis	
Reduction ⟷	No consistent change
Conjugation	
Microsomal enzyme activity ↓	Induction effects ↓
Renal clearance ↓ **	Blood levels ↑ e.g. digoxin,
	antidepressants, sulphas, thiazides,
	aminoglycosides
Pharmacodynamics	
Brain sensitivity ↑	Response to psychosedative drugs ↑ e.g.
	benzodiazepines, anticholinergics,
	opiates
Coagulation mechanism control ↓	Response to warfarin ↑
Adrenergic receptor sensitivity ↓	Responses to both agonists and
	antagonists ↓

*Increased absorption may be due to other mechanisms, e.g. levodopa ↑ because gastric decarboxylase ↓ and drug availability ↑
**The single most important kinetic factor
Key: ↓ = decrease ↑ = increase ⟷ = no significant or consistent change

these questions early and unless the outcomes are particularly clear a series of options should be considered ranging from the best to the worst clinical and social scenarios.

Geriatric pharmacology

The most pertinent age changes affecting drug treatment are shown in Table 20.1. Even more important than age with respect to safety and efficacy of drugs are:

1 The presence of disease, occult or manifest which may affect both clearance and response to drugs. For example, both factors are highly relevant to the use of digoxin but not of penicillin.

2 The use of polypharmacy leading to adverse drug-drug interactions. These are most likely when drugs are given in combination with others that have a narrow therapeutic index such as anticoagulants, antidepressants, anticonvulsants, antihypertensives, oral hypoglycaemic agents, cardiac glycosides and cytotoxic agents.

It is necessary to consider all aspects of the use of drugs by the patient because quite often it is broader issues, rather than 'pure' clinical pharmacology, which determine the outcome. The chain of events is—prescription, administration, pharmacokinetics, pharmacodynamics, with the clinical response largely dependent upon multiple factors including: ageing, accumulated pathology, concurrent drug use, the patient's behaviour and especially her interactions with friends, family and health and social services.

Drug use by the elderly

There is evidence of extensive use and misuse of drugs by elderly people in the UK. Those aged 65 plus (about 15 per cent of the population) are prescribed about a third of all medicines, additionally:

● Age 75+, 70–80 per cent of people are taking prescribed medicines, mostly as long-term repeats.

● More than one-third of females are taking long-term psychotropic medication.

● Age 65+ about one-third of all prescribed medicines appear to be unnecessary or at best of doubtful value in a pharmacological sense, especially tranquillizers, hypnotics, antidepressants, digoxin, diuretics and hypotensive agents.

● 25–30 per cent of this age group also self-medicate using over-the-counter medicine, e.g. for pain, coughs, colds and constipation.

Effective prescribing

The aim is to provide maximum benefit with minimum hazard. Many problems brought to the doctor are not amenable to drug treatment but may be helped by the adoption of a modified lifestyle with respect to diet, alcohol and physical exercise and the use of mechanical devices such as walking aids and household adaptations and the acceptance of social support. It is necessary to invest time and patience fully to understand the patient's medical problems and to decide what might be achieved by drug treatment. Prioritization of the treatable may be necessary for it is rarely useful or practicable to attempt to prescribe a pill for every ill. The essentials of effective prescribing are:

1 Make a full diagnosis and aim at key problems in order of priority.
2 Consider the effects of organ failure and any likely drug-drug interactions.
3 With drugs possessed of a low therapeutic index, and when clearance may be reduced, start with the lowest possible dose and cautiously increase.
4 Prescribe only drugs with which you are familiar; keep the drug list short and simple in its timing, e.g. twice rather than 4 times daily.
5 Monitor compliance and response.
6 At review stage, stop drugs no longer strictly indicated and always discard a drug to make way for a new prescription.

Drug administration and compliance

More than 90 per cent of the medicines consumed by the elderly in the UK are formulated as pills (tablets or capsules). These are generally much more convenient than liquid preparations such as mixtures or elixirs. The pills are most readily swallowed with food and drink at mealtimes. Important exceptions are the hypoglycaemic agents and some antibiotics (e.g. tetracyclines, but not doxycycline or minocycline) which should be taken 30 minutes before food or a milk drink.

The fairly common complaint of the pills 'sticking' should be taken seriously by the doctor because delayed pill-oesophageal-transit time is very common even in those with normal oesophageal motility as judged by radiology. Delay allows disintegration of the pill (especially capsules) within the oesophagus with the risk of ulceration, usually at the lower end but occasionally at the level of the left main-stem bronchus. To prevent 'sticking', pills should be swallowed in the upright, sitting or standing position and washed down with at least 50–60 ml of liquid (preferably twice as much). For 'bedtime' drugs, allow a minimum of 10–15 minutes before recumbency. Occasionally a switch to a liquid preparation proves to be necessary but the mode of administration should be as stated above.

Compliance
Compliance is the extent to which the patient adheres to the doctor's prescription whether it be for pill-taking or modification of lifestyle. Assuming accurate diagnosis, and the selection of an appropriate medicine and formulation, thought must be given to the degree of compliance required and how it is to be achieved. At home or in the hospital, it cannot be assumed that the medicine will be taken just as the doctor prescribes it. Fortunately the precise time of administration is not critical for most drugs although there are some important exceptions as for example levodopa in the later stages of Parkinson's disease. The patient and probably her carers should be trained in the management of the medicines. The task must be made as simple as possible and use made of memory aids and appropriate containers. Estimates of the prevalence of non-compliance vary enormously but around one-third is usual and the major causes appear to be:

1 Poor motivation
Patient asymptomatic or sees no reason for drugs.
Dislike or anxiety with respect to the immediate or long-term effects of the medicine.

2 Lack of understanding
A complex regimen, forgetfulness, running out of supply.

3 Practical problems
Dislike of formulation (taste, size, 'sticking'), impaired vision or manual dexterity, e.g. liquid medicines and inhalers.

4 Intelligent non-compliance
Patient decides risk or inconvenience not worthwhile (defence against the doctor).

Factors improving compliance

1 A simple, frugal treatment plan understood and agreed to by the patient.

2 In a stable situation, combinations and sustained release preparations can be used to reduce the number of pills to be taken. Three or four different preparations is about as many as most people can manage.

3 Simple, large-type script of the essential instructions.

4 Use of memory aids and cueing (see below).

5 Positive involvement of carers.

6 Clear-cut benefits from the medicine.

Taking the pills at mealtimes or just before bedtime provides useful cues and, if necessary, a separate container can be pre-loaded for each occasion. Alternatively compartmentalized day- or week-boxes (e.g. Dosett box or Pillwheel) may be used in the same way. Medicines to be taken at other times require their own special cues, e.g. an alarm clock or watch. It can be valuable to have an example of each pill, fixed to a piece of white card with sellotape, alongside the instructions (see Fig. 20.1). Patient package-inserts help the patient to know more about her medicines (if she can read the small

The tablets	Names and strengths	Purpose	To be taken
○	Digoxin 125 mcg	heart	1 at breakfast
⊕	Navidrex 500 mcg (cyclopenthiazide)	water	" " "
⬭	Sinemet–Plus	Parkinson's	" " "
	Sinemet–Plus	"	1 at lunch
	Sinemet–Plus	"	1 at supper
⊘	Amitriptyline 25 mg	nerves	1 with drink ½ hour before bed

Fig. 20.1. Medication display chart.

print) and may provide some legal cover for the prescriber and manufacturer, but they must not take the place of the doctor's own explanations.

Review of prescriptions

Follow-up by the family doctor is essential for the patient on long-term medication but the frequency of review will depend upon the need, for instance:

- Control of a newly diagnosed diabetic or patient with heart failure—daily.
- Maintenance treatment of the stable diabetic or heart failure patient—3–4 monthly.
- Maintenance of corrected hypothyroidism or pernicious anaemia—annually.

At review, other aspects of the patient's health and welfare should also be considered. A card index or computerized recall system is required to stop patients 'falling through the net'. Repeat prescriptions without appropriate medical review are both wasteful and hazardous. The number of repeat prescriptions between consultations has to be decided for each individual patient taking into account personality, the disease, the drug and the likely response.

Adverse effects (AEs) of drugs

Adverse effects or adverse drug reactions are at least twice as common in the elderly as in the young. The incidence rises with both age and the number of drugs prescribed. Most drugs have not yet had their pharmacology critically assessed in elderly subjects. Until this occurs, prescribing must be an uncertain activity and caution the watchword:

1 More than 20 per cent of patients aged 75 years and over, taking prescribed medicines during a single stay in hospital or during treatment at home, will experience a clinically significant adverse reaction to drugs.

2 In general medical wards, 10 per cent of the elderly patients are there directly or indirectly, because of AEs.

3 In geriatric wards, where the average age of 'the elderly' is much higher, AEs occur in around 15 per cent of those taking up to 3 different drugs and 20 per cent of those taking 4 or more preparations
daily.

4 Elderly patients are especially liable to suffer mental confusion, impaired psychomotor reactions, falls, postural hypotension and marrow toxicity as a result of drug treatment.

5 Drugs most often implicated are diuretics (relatively 'safe' but so extensively and often unnecessarily used), digoxin, psychotropic drugs, anti-Parkinsonian agents, hypotensives and antidiabetic drugs.

6 Adverse effects may be readily recognizable, e.g. hypoglycaemia with antidiabetics or bleeding with anticoagulants. Other AEs may be mistaken for illness, e.g. anorexia or increasing oedema with an anti-inflammatory agent or may be missed altogether as with a failed response to an oral penicillin given concurrently with oral iron.

7 Many factors other than those due to ageing contribute to the high incidence of adverse drug reactions in elderly patients, particularly:

- Multimorbidity and the inevitable polypharmacy it invites.
- Uncritical assessment of the need for drug treatment.
- Prescribing without due regard to concurrent medications.

Surgical treatment

Age itself should be no bar to surgery; with modern techniques 85 per cent of elderly patients with surgical problems can be given more or less complete relief and a further 10 per cent partial relief. Much of the excess post-operative morbidity and mortality of the elderly relates to coincidental medical illness rather than simply to age or the stress of the operation. Currently, in UK general hospitals:

- Surgeons admit as many elderly patients as general physicians and geriatricians combined.
- 25 per cent of patients admitted to surgical beds are age 65 and over and about 10 per cent are age 75 and over.
- In orthopaedics the admission rate almost doubles decade by decade over the age of 65.
- In ophthalmology and urology about 50 per cent cases are age 65 and over.
- The general elective surgery post-operative mortality rate is less than 5 per cent if the likely 'non-viable' cases (e.g. advanced cancer) are excluded.

• Emergency surgery is particularly hazardous in the elderly, e.g. elective cholecystectomy operative mortality less than 2 per cent and emergency cholecystectomy mortality 20–30 per cent.

• Potentially preventable or treatable causes of death are heart failure, myocardial infarction, pneumonia, pulmonary embolism, stroke and a few technical surgical complications.

Pre-operative assessment

The pre-operative assessment should include a careful search for treatable concomitant medical conditions, a judgement regarding the most appropriate premedication and time to develop rapport between the anaesthetist and the patient; the assessment is performed by the surgical team and the anaesthetist. The contribution of the geriatrician can be valuable in selected cases regarding the medical aspects of management, post-operative rehabilitation and relocation at home or elsewhere. This is especially true in orthopaedics where a good working relationship with geriatric medicine is highly desirable. Elderly patients must be handled physically and pharmacologically with great care because:

• The skin is usually thin and liable to tear, e.g. when pulling off sticking plaster or pulling the sheets from under the patient—lift her!

• Haematoma readily follows venepuncture—elevate the arm and maintain pressure over the puncture site.

• Stiff joints may limit surgical access; stiff necks must not be forced into 'normal' alignment!

• Time is needed pre-operatively to bring medical illness under control, to allow slow induction of anaesthesia and to reverse the effects of the anaesthetic especially muscle-paralysing agents e.g. tubocurarine.

• There is enhanced sensitivity to CNS depressant drugs—scale down doses of anaesthetic agents, benzodiazepines and opioid analgesics.

In the routine checking of the patient pay specific attention to:

1 Treatable conditions such as anaemia, volume depletion, heart failure and respiratory infection.

2 Assessment of the mental state pre-operatively and over the preceding months as reported by the carers—is the patient dementing? An acute confusional state is most likely to be due to drugs or acute illness but there may be underlying dementia.

3 Abuse of alcohol and tobacco, problems with dietary intake and recent weight loss. Beware of withdrawal syndromes with respect to alcohol and drugs, e.g. hypnotics, narcotics, antidepressants, anticonvulsants, anti-Parkinsonians, beta-blockers, calcium antagonists and corticosteroids.

4 Assessment of pre-morbid physical capabilities and the need for social support—think in terms of eventual discharge from day one! Ideally this should be done prior to admission for surgery.

5 Routine chest X–ray and ECG which are valuable for detection of unsuspected pathology and for comparison post-operatively, if complications develop.

Pre-operative preparation

The time allowed will be determined by surgical urgency:

1 Correct salt and water depletion to help maintain BP and renal function and even if patient appears stable repeat the urea and electrolytes on the third or fourth post-operative day.

2 Correct moderate to severe anaemia by transfusion, if speed is of the essence.

3 Treat heart failure and respiratory infection and cover ethanol withdrawal with chlormethiazole orally and Parentrovite parenterally.

4 Improve nutrition if there is evidence of markedly reduced food intake in the preceding weeks or months, sudden weight loss or protein malnutrition, e.g. little muscle mass and serum albumin level of less than 28 g/l. Nasogastric feeding or parenteral alimentation may be required.

5 If time allows, delay operation to correct gross obesity and strengthen muscles to reduce the risk of post-operative pneumonia and wound complications; moderate obesity can be ignored.

Post-operative complications

1 Respiratory

Post-operative respiratory infections account for 20–40 per cent of all complications and one-sixth to one-third of all post-operative deaths in the over 65s. The usual cause is small airways closure leading to atelectasis and pneumonia. This is due to suppression of sustained maximal inspirations or 'sighs' by sedation or pain especially with an incision near to the diaphragm. The elderly are much more likely to be affected than the young. Additional risk

factors for post-operative chest infections are:
- Pre-operative chest disease.
- Volume depletion (dehydration).
- Cigarette smoking.
- Severe obesity.

Prevention of post-operative chest complications:
- Stop smoking.
- Reduce weight.
- Deep breathing.
- Avoid over-sedation.

2 Cardiovascular

Congestive cardiac failure occurs in some 5–10 per cent and myocardial infarction in 1–3 per cent of elderly post-operative patients. Since at least 50 per cent of the infarctions are painless it is good practice, if things are not going well post-operatively, to have repeat ECGs to compare with the pre-operative record. Also look for clinical and radiological signs of congestive failure which may be precipitated by iv fluid overload. This is especially liable to occur on account of compromised renal function and reduced mechanical efficiency of the heart due to valvular disease, ischaemia, fibrosis or amyloid. A spell of O_2 therapy is often needed post-operatively to compensate for reduced PaO_2 due to the combined effects of ageing, hypoventilation and ventilation/perfusion abnormalities. Cold surgery should be delayed for at least 3 months after myocardial infarction.

3 Stroke

The incidence of post-operative stroke is about 1 per cent over age 65 and 3 per cent over age 80 years. Surprisingly previous stroke or the presence of a carotid bruit appears not to increase the risk of post-operative stroke. It is generally advised to postpone an operation for 2–3 months after a stroke. Because of the prevalence of impaired cerebrovascular autoregulation in the elderly (and especially in those with cerebrovascular disease), wide swings of blood pressure are to be avoided.

4 Acute confusional states

Emergence delirium on waking from the anaesthetic is no more common in the elderly than in the young whereas interval delirium coming on later in the first week is much more common with an

incidence of 10–15 per cent in the over 65s. Delirium tremens is occasionally seen. Interval delirium is the major problem and the likely causes are:
• Hypoxia, fluid and electrolyte imbalance.
• Physical disease especially respiratory infection and heart failure.
• Unrelieved distress from the operation wound, distended viscus and pressure areas.
• Sedative and psychotropic drugs.
Simply to sedate the acutely confused patient will make matters worse; treatment of the underlying causes almost always makes things better.

5 Deep vein thrombosis and pulmonary embolism
Research using radio-isotope labelled fibrinogen scanning or phlebography has shown that deep vein thrombosis (DVT) occurs in between a quarter and a third of all general surgical patients over the age of 40 years and that the risk increases with age. Further increases in risk relate to pelvic or hip surgery and to the use of general anaesthesia as opposed to epidural or spinal analgesia. Other risk factors for DVT and pulmonary embolus are:
• Previous history of thromboembolic disease.
• Prolonged immobility and dehydration.
• Severe obesity and trauma to calves.
• Malignancy.
• Cardiorespiratory disease.
• Oestrogen therapy.

Prevention
• Low-dose heparin given subcutaneously appears to be effective in general surgical cases but not in operations on the hip.
• Other methods advocated but not proven, include: pneumatic compression of the calves, regular ankle flexion-extension movements throughout the peri-operative period, graded pressure stockings, full anti-coagulation, aspirin and dextran.

Further reading
Black D. (1984) Medication for the elderly. A report of the Royal College of Physicians. *Journal of the Royal College of Physicians*, **18**, 7–17.
Caird F.I. (1985) Towards rational drug therapy in old age. *Journal of The Royal College of Physicians*, **19**, 235–9.

Consumer's Association (1984) Surgery and long-term medication. *Drug and Therapeutics Bulletin,* **22,** 73–6.

Dodson M.E. (1987) Aspects of anaesthesia in the elderly. *British Journal of Hospital Medicine,* **37,** 114–20

George C.F. (1985) Hazards of the abrupt withdrawal of drugs. *Prescribers Journal,* **25,** 31–9.

Seymour D.G. & Vaz F.G. (1987) Aspects of surgery in the elderly: pre-operative medical assessment. *British Journal of Hospital Medicine,* **37,** 102–12.

Chapter 21
Death and Dying

Ageing and death

Ageing may be regarded as an increasing inability to resist death. In the UK people are least liable to die around the age of puberty. Thereafter, age-specific death rates increase more and more rapidly, see Fig. 21.1. Almost 80 per cent of UK deaths occur in those aged 65 years and over and in women almost 65 per cent of deaths are in those aged 75 years and over. In the UK most deaths occur in institutions especially in National Health Service (NHS) hospitals (see Table 21.1). The most common causes of death in elderly people are shown in Table 21.2.

Pre-death dependence has serious implications for patient and family. Although most people die in hospital the terminal phase of life can be a very protracted affair with increased dependence on family, friends and others for many months or even years. This, coupled with possible loss of mental faculties and an associated lack of dignity, is a dreaded prospect. More than anything else it feeds the desire for 'some other way' such as voluntary euthanasia. Elderly people have had ample time to come to terms with their own

Table 21.1. Place of death, all causes, all ages in England and Wales 1985

Location	Male %	Female %
NHS hospitals	58	59
(includes psychiatric)	(1.7)	(2.2)
All other institutions	7	14
Deceased person's home	28	23
Other places	7	4
Total deaths	292 327	298 407

(Adapted from OPCS data)

230

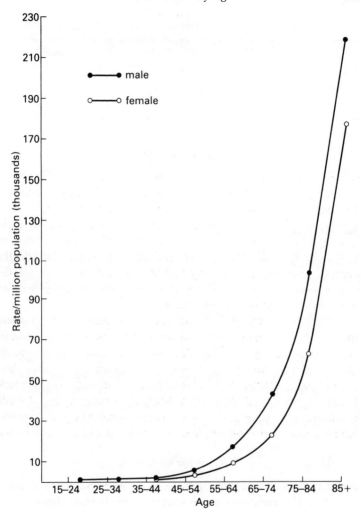

Fig. 21.1. Age-specific death rates, all causes England 1985, adapted from OPCS data Table 13, DHI no. 17.

mortality and are readily able to accept the prospect of death. What they fear at the end is the mode of dying and 'being a nuisance'.

Management of death and dying

Death and dying is of major concern to those who care for the elderly. We must be aware of the needs both of the dying person and

Table 21.2. The five most common causes of death in the aged in England, 1985

Cause of death (ICD Numbers)	SMR approx. rates/1000	Males			Females		
		65–74, years	75–84, years	85+ years	65–74, years	75–84, years	85+ years
Ischaemic heart disease (410–414)	97	15.4	30.4	51.8	6.7	17.3	39.0
Diseases of the respiratory system (460–519)	97	4.5	14.9	46.9	1.8	6.0	27.7
Cerebrovascular disease (430–438)	97	3.9	12.8	29.9	2.9	11.5	33.0
Neoplasms (140–239)	100	13.2	23.9	32.7	7.6	11.7	18.0
Diseases of the digestive system, non-neoplastic 520–579)	99	1.0	2.7	6.7	0.8	2.3	6.8

ICD = International classification of diseases; SMR = Standardized mortality ratio, all ages, UK = 100 (adapted from OPCS data).

of her supporting relatives and friends. Honesty, sensitivity and tact are always desirable but especially in 'paving the last mile'. The final illness offers an opportunity for the family to come together and develop socially, emotionally and spiritually; this brings solace to both patient and relatives and it facilitates bereavement.

Plans for home care

In the period of increasing pre-death dependence and well before the stage of terminal care it is necessary to alleviate those stresses which are found to be least tolerable to the patient and her supporters, for example:
- Sleep disturbance.
- Urinary incontinence.
- Restricted social life of the key carers.
- Immobility.
- Faecal incontinence.

These common serious problems listed in order of prevalence in pre-death dependence and terminal care are referred to in other chapters. The first and last are particularly ill tolerated but all are important, and there may well be others such as unrelieved pain or mental confusion. It is vital not to be lulled into a false sense of security when people struggle with burdens such as these. Eventually they crack and the patient may spend an unnecessarily long time in hospital as a result. It is better to forestall the breakdown in home care by early recognition and positive management of strain.

Role of the general practitioner
The general practitioner acts as physician, confidant, counsellor and orchestrator of help from a wide range of sources:

1 Informal help
Relatives and friends, clergy and voluntary agencies such as Age Concern.

2 Help from health and social services
Home nursing, home help, laundry service, financial assistance, e.g. constant attendance allowance and supplementary benefit.

Family resources should be augmented progressively to allow home care to continue. As the terminal phase draws near it might be necessary to increase the amount of support beyond that available from the statutory services. Extra nursing and domestic help may be obtained from private or voluntary agencies.

Involvement of the geriatrician
If there is doubt about the home-care programme early domiciliary consultation with the geriatrician is indicated. In addition to an appraisal of the medical aspects of the case he can review the care plans, meet the key carers and help to decide between home and hospital. Close collaboration between the community nurse and the geriatric liaison health visitor is valuable in sorting out the practical arrangements. A short spell of inpatient care may be indicated to bring symptoms under control, to work out the most appropriate drug schedule and to firm up the clinical diagnosis. Later there can be planned, or occasionally urgent, re-admission to allow relatives respite. The aim is to allow all parties involved (carers and cared for) to receive practical help and emotional support with due regard to what is available locally.

Management of anxiety

Anxiety in the patient and all those in contact with her is a major problem in the period of pre-death dependence and in terminal care. The main causes are:

(i) *Worry about diagnostic or treatment error*—relatives need to be assured that no curative options remain.

(ii) *Uncertainty about process*—'What happens if?' the relatives ask. They need to be reassured that practical problems can be dealt with, e.g. pain, vomiting, falls and incontinence; unrelieved pain is especially anxiety provoking.

(iii) *Feelings of inadequacy*—often the carers imagine that the patient would receive more and better quality attention in hospital. Occasionally this is true, but often it is not because the hospital cannot possibly know and accommodate the patient's idiosyncracies as her intimates do. Furthermore home care may be on the basis of one patient to one attendant for much of the 24 hours. In hospital the patient will have to share the attention of the nurses on duty with many others.

(iv) *Ambivalent attitudes*—are common in patient and relatives with, for example, vacillation between the need to know and preferring not to know the diagnosis or the urge to 'get it all over with' and yet feeling guilty to entertain such thoughts.

Telling the patient

The question 'Am I about to die?' will often be on the patient's mind for weeks or months before she dares to put it into words. Spending time with the patient, preferably in private, will allow the question to be asked. When it comes it is not to be brushed aside nor should a trite answer be given. If there is doubt as to what to say it is better simply to keep the conversation going and give the patient the opportunity to talk about problems which worry her most. Lies are never required. The patient who really wishes to know should be told clearly, simply and with compassion while giving room for hope and the assurance that the doctor will not abandon her and that suffering will be relieved.

Symptom control in terminal care

General principles

1 Symptom control becomes paramount when there is no hope of cure or worthwhile remission.

2 Allow the patient to live her life to the full, devoid of irksome restrictions and with optimal cerebration.

3 Adopt a broad but meticulous approach to the analysis of the patient's distress because each and every discomfort exacerbates the total pain.

4 Symptoms may not be due to the main illness but to:
- Complications such as constipation or pressure sores.
- Coexisting disease such as cardiac failure or pneumonia.
- Medical treatment, e.g. drips, injections or drugs causing nausea and vomiting.

5 Arrange good nursing care with special attention to personal hygiene including care of the mouth, adequate hydration, comfortable clean clothing and bed.

6 Encourage reliable, compatible companionship; patient requires time alone but not so much as to be lonely.

Mental symptoms

Anxiety, insomnia and depression
Provided that all practical measures have been taken to relieve physical and social distress then use of minor tranquillizers, hypnotics or antidepressants as appropriate will be indicated.

Restlessness and confusion
Physical discomfort and illness can be a major precipitant; for example an overloaded bladder or rectum or an infection in the chest or urinary tract. Treatment of the cause will obviate the need to increase the dose of tranquillizer. If restlessness and agitation persist, use of a major tranquillizer will be justified, parenterally if necessary.

Physical symptoms

Pain, mild to moderate
Some pain is common in the terminal illness. The aim is to secure pain control throughout the 24 hours. Start with paracetamol or aspirin every 4 hours and gradually increase the dose to achieve control. Some patients do better with a compound preparation such as co-codaprin or co-proxamol but the opiate will constipate and in bigger doses cause drowsiness. NSAIDs are also useful here.

Pain, moderate to severe
Severe, intractable pain is mercifully rare in the elderly person facing death. When it occurs strong analgesics are required especially morphia or heroin every 4 hours by mouth, rectum or parenterally; laxatives will then be necessary. Morphine sulphate controlled-release tablets need to be given only twice daily. The analgesic can be topped up if necessary with aspirin, paracetamol or NSAIDs. Continuous subcutaneous infusion of diamorphine (and other drugs) by syringe driver offers a comfortable alternative to repeated intramuscular injections. Headache from raised intracranial pressure may be relieved by use of dexamethasone. Prednisolone eases general malaise.

Gastrointestinal symptoms
For anorexia, nausea and vomiting consider the possibility of an iatrogenic cause. Otherwise use a major tranquillizer such as chlorpromazine and possibly metoclopramide. If severe abdominal pain and vomiting are due to intestinal obstruction, even in far-advanced malignant disease, the surgeon should be consulted because, there may be a non-malignant cause and other causes may be relieved for several months by operation. If surgery is not indicated it is better not to persist with 'drip and suck' but to ablate the symptoms with drugs:
• Intestinal colic—use smooth muscle relaxants such as loperamide, hyoscine or atropine.
• Vomiting—use phenothiazines especially chlorpromazine or prochlorperazine, orally when vomiting is intermittent, otherwise by rectal suppositories or intramuscularly.
• Abdominal pain not due to colic—use analgesics as described above.
• Diarrhoea—use codeine or loperamide.

Respiratory symptoms
Cough usually responds to diamorphine linctus and breathlessness to morphine and oxygen although some patients cannot tolerate the mask. The 'death rattle' is usually relieved by hyoscine or atropine, but with the risk of the central anticholinergic syndrome of agitation, hallucinations and dysphoria.

Skin symptoms
Pruritus from cholestasis may respond to chlorpromazine or

fluoxymesterone. Capillary bleeding from a fungating growth can be treated with adrenaline 1 in 1000 solution applied on a piece of gauze, and smell from the ulcer reduced by means of mild antiseptic soaks and cleansing agents.

After death

After death a doctor should see the body to confirm and certify death. The death must be registered within 5 days at the local sub-district office of the Registrar of Births and Deaths. Patients dying soon after admission to hospital (within 24 hours), and where the cause of death is believed to be natural, should have the death certificate completed by the family doctor, otherwise it is best to inform the coroner.

The coroner

If the cause of death is unknown, occurs in suspicious circumstances or has an unnatural cause, the coroner must be consulted immediately and if there is to be an enquiry the relatives should be informed of the implications without delay. If the coroner accepts the case, the body becomes the property of the Crown and cannot be disposed of or tampered with without his permission. If the coroner requires an autopsy this can be done even against the expressed wishes of the deceased, the relatives or any religious beliefs. An inquest may be held if death was thought to be unnatural and there may or may not be a jury depending on the nature of the case. After the autopsy the body is usually released to the family for burial or cremation but at this stage the findings of the autopsy may not necessarily be disclosed. Only the coroner may authorize cremation in these cases.

Deaths to report to the coroner

The doctor must exercise his judgement in individual cases, but when in doubt ring the coroner's office. The following should be reported:

1 Accident, misadventure, starvation, severe deprivation (neglect), poisoning.

2 Drugs, therapeutic or of addiction or abuse including alcoholism.

3 Anaesthetics, surgical or medical mishap, and also when relatives express serious dissatisfaction or allege neglect.

4 Industrial disease, even if not a cause of death.

5 Septicaemia of possible unnatural cause.
6 Those with disability pensions from service with the Crown.
7 Prisoners and anyone in the custody of the police.

Preservation of evidence
Since deaths in suspicious circumstances may lead to criminal or civil proceedings material taken from the patient, e.g. drugs, clothing, gastric washings and flakes of paint should be carefully noted and preserved. Meticulous documentation of wounds, bruises, marks, etc. and statements by the patient regarding the circumstances of the injuries, can be immensely important.

Bereavement

The prevalence of widowhood increases rapidly after middle age. In Britain whereas only 2 per cent of men and 8 per cent of women aged between 45 and 59 are widowed this increases to 30 per cent of men and 64 per cent of women among those age 75 and over.

The loss of a near and dear one, especially a spouse or child, precipitates serious but entirely normal emotional reactions of intense grief. Similar reactions may occur after other losses which are particularly hard to bear such as amputation of a limb, loss of fortune or self-esteem or the break-up of a marriage. These losses are not only more common than bereavement but may be more severe because they are perceived to be out of the natural order of things and the victim finds it very hard to adjust.

Grief reactions
Five phases of grief have been described in bereavement:

1 Denial and isolation. The disbelief may last for hours or days. The bereaved simply cannot accept what has happened and is emotionally and intellectually blunted.

2 Anger towards self or others. It is often the doctor or other carer who bears the brunt, and who must soak up the invective of the attack. He must respond with extreme tact and sensitivity, listening rather than talking back, showing no anger and attempting no rebuttal. This phase may be combined with phase 3.

3 Bargaining for a better deal. Seen also in anticipatory grief. Promises are given of changed behaviour if there can be another chance. May have illusions of the presence of the deceased in sight, sound or touch. These two phases last for days or weeks.

4 Mental depression. The loss is now accepted but life is not worth living. A phase of physiological depression with a flat, lacklustre mood. This is normal, it passes off with time but may take months.

5 Acceptance. The survivor is now prepared to carry on and return to normal life. This may take 1–2 years and the bereaved is a changed person after these highly charged emotional experiences.

Anticipatory grief
When the death can be foreseen, grieving begins early and this is important because it allows both the dying person and the family to prepare for the future. By working through unfinished business, making contingency plans and grieving together (sometimes angrily) the eventual death and bereavement will be a much less traumatic experience. Sudden, unexpected death does not allow this to happen and the reaction is thus more likely to be profound or pathological.

Pathological grief
An abnormal grief pattern may be observed where the bereaved person:
- Suffers excessively high levels of anxiety and may even become psychotic.
- Is stuck in the grieving process for an abnormally long time and clearly 'can't get over it'.
- Experiences extreme feelings of guilt; may be ambivalent about the death being glad that 'it is all over' and then is filled with remorse, self-reproach and despair.

The grief reaction can be catastrophic and a major risk factor for suicide especially in the elderly, socially isolated male. Pathological grief occurs notably following sudden or untimely deaths and when blame could attach to the survivor. It also has much to do with:
- The quality of the relationship, being more likely with loss of a spouse or where the relationship was unusually close or dependent.
- The personality of the survivor, some people being particularly grief prone, clinging and insecure or who already have much stress

to cope with on account of serious mental or physical illness or disability.

• Social factors including lack of close support from friends, family, church or employment, low socioeconomic status and a series of bereavements or other severe stresses in a short period of time.

Management of grief
This is essentially a human rather than a medical problem. Nevertheless the doctor will almost certainly be consulted at some stage, and there may be requests for 'medical treatment' for the bereavement reactions. In the main these should be resisted. Time, tea and sympathy are the great healers here, not modern pharmaceuticals.

An urgent requirement is for a friend or relative to take over the household, register the death and make the funeral arrangements. Also the bereaved needs someone 'to be there', someone to talk to, a listener who does not necessarily wish to talk back, someone who will accept and gently reassure. It there is much anger and depression there is the danger that the very people who could help may be driven away. Family, friends, care practitioners and voluntary helpers must not allow themselves to indulge in avoidance behaviour on account of these difficulties. Spiritual help can be valuable later even for erstwhile disbelievers! Sleeping pills and tranquillizers are not to be used except possibly very short term and intermittently. An antidepressant may occasionally be valuable. Help may also come from Age Concern or the social services through bereavement counselling (listening, reassuring, counselling). Similarly the voluntary society CRUSE will use local contacts to befriend the bereaved.

People are needed to stay around long after the funeral to absorb the anger and despair of the bereaved. All must adopt a waiting and watching role and not try to hasten the grieving process. Unless there are compelling reasons to the contrary, decisions regarding moving house or living with relatives should be arrived at when the emotional torment has subsided rather than early in bereavement. For the more intractable grief reactions, psychotherapy or specific 'guided' grieving techniques may be required. Eventually, the bereaved must say a final 'goodbye' to the lost partner and build a new life.

Medical implications of bereavement

Recent bereavement and relocation of the elderly are associated with increased morbidity and mortality from a wide range of disorders. Because of this the doctor should keep in touch to permit early intervention if things go wrong. The reasons for the excess illness are not satisfactorily explained but possibilities include loss of care and companionship ('loneliness can damage, if not break the human heart'), personal neglect and stress-induced neuroendocrine changes. Furthermore it is not uncommon for people to take ill or at least consult the doctor at or around the anniversary of death of a spouse or other major loss. These dates should be noted in the clinical record so that the significance of the visit is seen in context. The care of the survivors goes on.

Further reading

McAvoy B.R. (1986) Death after bereavement. *British Medical Journal*, **293**, 835.

Stott N.C. (1986) Easing progress through the five stages of bereavement. *Geriatric Medicine*, **16**, 24–6.

Twycross R.G. (1986) Care of the dying: symptom control. *British Journal of Hospital Medicine*, **36**, 244–9.

Index